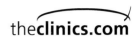
theclinics.com

NURSING CLINICS
OF NORTH AMERICA

Perioperative Nursing

GUEST EDITOR
Gratia M. Nagle, RN, BA, CNOR, CRNFA,
CRLS, CURN

June 2006 • Volume 41 • Number 2

SAUNDERS

An Imprint of Elsevier, Inc.
PHILADELPHIA   LONDON   TORONTO   MONTREAL   SYDNEY   TOKYO

W.B. SAUNDERS COMPANY
A Division of Elsevier Inc.

1600 John F. Kennedy Blvd., Suite 1800, Philadelphia, PA 19103-2899

http://www.theclinics.com

NURSING CLINICS OF NORTH AMERICA	Volume 41, Number 2
June 2006	ISSN 0029-6465
Editor: Ali Gavenda	ISBN 1-4160-3535-4

The ideas and opinions expressed in *Nursing Clinics of North America* do not necessarily reflect those of the Publisher. The Publisher does not assume any responsibility for any injury and/or damage to persons or property arising out of or related to any use of the material contained in this periodical. The reader is advised to check the appropriate medical literature and the product information currently provided by the manufacturer of each drug to be administered to verify the dosage, the method and duration of administration, or contraindications. It is the responsibility of the treating physician or other health care professional, relying on independent experience and knowledge of the patient, to determine drug dosages and the best treatment for the patient. Mention of any product in this issue should not be construed as endorsement by the contributors, editors, or the Publisher of the product or manufacturers' claims.

Nursing Clinics of North America (ISSN 0029-6465) is published quarterly by W.B. Saunders, 360 Park Avenue South, New York, NY 10010-1710. Months of publication are March, June, September, and December. Business and Editorial Offices: 1600 John F. Kennedy Blvd., Suite 1800, Philadelphia, PA 19103-2899. Accounting and Circulation Offices: 6277 Sea Harbor Drive, Orlando, FL 32887-4800. Periodicals postage paid at New York, NY and additional mailing offices. Subscription price per year is, $105.00 (US individuals), $200.00 (US institutions), $170.00 (international individuals), $240.00 (international institutions), $145.00 (Canadian individuals), $240.00 (Canadian institutions), $55.00 (US students), and $85.00 (international students). To receive student/resident rate, orders must be accompanied by name of affiliated institution, date of term, and the signature of program/residency coordinator on institution letterhead. Orders will be billed at individual rate until proof of status is received. Foreign air speed delivery is included in all *Clinics* subscription prices. All prices are subject to change without notice. **POSTMASTER:** Send address changes to *Nursing Clinics of North America*, Elsevier Periodicals Customer Service, 6277 Sea Harbor Drive, Orlando, FL 32887-4800. **Customer Service: 1-800-654-2452 (US). From outside of the US, call 1-407-345-4000.**

Nursing Clinics of North America is covered in *EMBASE/Excerpta Medica, Index Medicus, Social Sciences Citation Index, Current Contents, ASCA, Cumulative Index to Nursing, RNdex Top 100*, and *Allied Health Literature and International Nursing Index (INI)*.

Printed in the United States of America.

NURSING CLINICS
OF NORTH AMERICA

Perioperative Nursing

GUEST EDITOR

GRATIA M. NAGLE, RN, BA, CNOR, CRNFA, CRLS, CURN, Paoli, Pennsylvania

CONTRIBUTORS

ANDREA BRAY, RN, MSN, CNOR, RNFA, Highlands Ranch, Colorado

PHYLLIS M. HOUCK, RN, MS HEd, CNOR, Staff Nurse/OR Educator, Operating Room, Paoli Hospital, Paoli, Pennsylvania

DOLLY IRELAND, MSN, RN, CAPA, CPN, Director of Education, Crittenton Hospital Medical Center, Rochester, Michigan; Adjunct Faculty, Oakland Community College, Highland Lakes, Waterford, Michigan

MYRNA EILEEN MAMARIL, MS, RN, CPAN, CAPA, Nurse Manager, Perianesthesia Services, University of Colorado Hospital, Denver, Colorado

MARY PATRICIA O'CONNELL, CRNA, Nurse Anesthetist, Paoli Hospital, Paoli, Pennsylvania

TRACY MARTINEZ OWENS, RN, BSN, Program Director, Wittgrove Bariatric Center, Scripps Memorial Hospital, La Jolla, California

DONNA M. DEFAZIO QUINN, BSN, MBA, RN, CPAN, CAPA, Director, Orthopaedic Surgery Center, Concord, New Hampshire

SHARON ROMANOSKI, RN, MBA, CNOR, RNFA, Operating Room Schedule Coordinator, Paoli Hospital, Paoli, Pennsylvania

DIANA L. WADLUND, RN, CRNFA, CRNP, Perioperative Nurse Practitioner, Surgical Specialists, West Chester, Pennsylvania

NURSING CLINICS
OF NORTH AMERICA

Perioperative Nursing

CONTENTS   VOLUME 41 • NUMBER 2 • JUNE 2006

Thorough assessment of the surgical patient begins in the preoperative phase and extends throughout the perioperative experience. Patient-centered interviews gather critical data that contribute to a successful experience and a focused plan of care. Information collected, documented, and conveyed to the surgeon or physician assists in appropriate medical decision making. This article focuses on perioperative nursing assessment tools and discusses issues pertinent to achieving safe delivery of care. A broad overview touches on key topics that deserve exploration and evaluation. This article will hopefully serve as a useful tool that helps direct the decision-making process.

A review of the literature focusing on postoperative complications reveals that the best available tools to the medical and surgical teams are recognition and prevention. This article highlights the more common postsurgical adverse events and discusses methods for preventing and treating these occurrences.

The operating room is unknown territory to most health care providers. It frequently brings up thoughts of blood, strange smells, and cold temperatures. Many nursing programs have scheduled little, if any, time in this environment for students. As a result, few nurses who practice outside of this specialized area understand the patient care events that occur in the operating room. Those who have selected the operating room for their work environment know that it is a somewhat isolated period in the perioperative experience. This article provides insight into this area of patient care and a greater understanding of how patients are positioned, the physiologic impact of these positions, and some consequences that may impact the postoperative care of these patients.

Although the discovery of laser light no longer can be termed recent, it took the medical community a long time to use its technology. Every day, advances are being made in laser technology, and new applications are being discovered for this modality. Because lasers allow for the capture, control, and manipulation of energy, it is important for nurses to understand the basic biophysics of lasers. As lasers are being used in most surgical settings and specialties, it is important for the perioperative nurse to have a basic knowledge of each wave length, type of laser, indications for its use, and safety considerations.

This article discusses the benefits and risks of laparoscopy. Also discussed are complications of laparoscopy and methods to avoid or treat these adversities.

Religion, language, and ethnicity play important roles in the perioperative arena. This article highlights some of the challenges that religion, language, and ethnicity can present and offers strategies for making the experience as positve as possible for all patients.

The American Society for Bariatric Surgery defines morbid obesity as a lifelong, progressive, life-threatening, genetically-related, costly, multifactorial disease of excess fat storage with multiple comorbidities. Obesity satisfies the definition of morbid obesity when it reaches the point of significant risk for obesity-related comorbidities. These significant comorbidities often result in either significant physical disability or even death. Obesity results from excessive accumulation of fat that exceeds the body skeletal and physical standards. Morbid obesity is defined as being at least 100 lb heavier than ideal body weight, or a body mass index (BMI) of 40. BMI is calculated as weight in kilograms divided by the height in meters squared. This article focuses on the causes, treatment, and perioperative nursing care of patients who are morbidly obese.

NURSING CLINICS
OF NORTH AMERICA

NURSING CLINICS
OF NORTH AMERICA

ELSEVIER
SAUNDERS

PREFACE

Perioperative Nursing

Gratia M. Nagle, RN, BA, CNOR, CRNFA, CRLS, CURN

Guest Editor

P erioperative nursing is not just "technical work anyone can do." Perioperative nurses are skilled, knowledgeable RNs who care for patients before, during, and after surgery. The fundamental nursing values (knowledge, skills, and judgment) are ever present and are the basis of the quality of care that surgical patients can expect and on which they can rely. We are no longer the "forgotten nurses," the mystical figures behind the operating room (OR) doors. People are being educated about what we do and see that we believe in what we are doing. We are..."A Tradition of Excellence" [1].

For the most part, nursing programs do not provide students with operating room experience. This is unfortunate because a comprehensive curriculum that offers perioperative nursing provides insight to and training in the surgical arena. In 1933, the National League for Nurses established a curriculum for schools of nursing that included courses in OR theory and clinical experience. The curriculum remained a model for training OR nurses until 1949, when the OR suddenly became the lowest priority [2]. The purpose of this issue of *Clinics* is to present issues that face perioperative nurses and the patients entrusted to their care. This issue contains topics that are hopefully of interest and relevant to all nurses involved in care of surgical patients.

I began working part time in the OR as a student nurse. Programs at that time provided the opportunity to take part in OR activities and perioperative patient care. I was fortunate enough to spend 3 months as a student in the OR and chose that specialty immediately after my clinical experience there. The nurses in the OR were called operating room nurses then. That terminology led to misconceptions about what exactly an operating room nurse did. We were often considered "not really nurses" because it was believed that what we did was purely technical in nature. Nothing could be farther from the truth.

A comprehensive introduction to the OR serves several purposes: (1) to provide a better understanding of the needs of surgical patients pre-, intra-, and postoperatively; (2) to provide insight into surgical interventions that can affect patient outcome directly; (3) to provide a chance for students to determine if this specialty area of nursing is something in which they might be competent

0029-6465/06/$ – see front matter
doi:10.1016/j.cnur.2006.02.001

and find enjoyment; and (4) to provide an opportunity to learn what perioperative nurses offer to nursing in general.

AORN (Association of periOperative Nurses) has developed specific guidelines, standards, and practice recommendations [3]. These guidelines are tempered by recommendations from Centers for Disease Control and Joint Commission for Accreditation of Health Care Organizations. Perioperative nurses have the opportunity to become certified after 2 years of experience (certified nurse operating room) and are encouraged to do so. Certified perioperative nurses have the opportunity to become a registered nurse first assistant through a didactic and clinical curriculum and obtain certification once entrance criteria have been met [4]. Many perioperative nurses also progress to advanced practice as certified registered nurse practitioners.

Just what is perioperative nursing? The first official statement that defined nursing care in the operating room was developed in 1969. AORN's current vision statement explains the term "perioperative nursing" as "the practice of nursing directed toward patients undergoing operative and other invasive procedures" [3]. The statement also defined this specialized nurse as "one who provides, manages, teaches, or studies the care of patients undergoing operative or other invasive procedures" [3].

Perioperative nurses are defined further by AORN in their perioperative patient-focused model as: "The registered nurse who, using the nursing process, develops a plan of nursing care and then coordinates and delivers care to patients undergoing operative and other invasive procedures. Perioperative nurses have the requisite skills and knowledge to assess, diagnose, plan, intervene, and evaluate the outcomes of interventions. The perioperative nurse addresses the physiological, psychological sociocultural, and spiritual responses of surgical patients" [3,5].

Perioperative nursing is one of the oldest nursing practices on record [2]. It can be traced back to 1875, when the first lecture was given to nurses at John Hopkins University. Florence Nightingale is considered the specialty's first and most distinguished practitioner [5,6]. The current AORN competency statements in perioperative nursing developed by the nursing practice committee revised the definition of perioperative nursing in 1984 to elaborate that "The registered nurse specializing in perioperative nursing practice performs nursing activities in the preoperative, intraoperative, and postoperative phases of the patient's surgical experience. Registered nurses enter perioperative nursing practice at a beginning level depending on their expertise and competency to practice. As they gain knowledge and skills, they progress on a continuum to an advanced level of practice" [3].

One might assume that these statements naturally would include any nurse involved in the care of surgical patients. In its broadest sense, perhaps. When the definition is reviewed, however, one sees that it is more circumscribed. Perioperative nurses may be generalists or specialize in a specific surgical specialty, such as orthopedics or open-heart surgery. Perioperative nurses new to the OR environment require an extensive orientation before they are considered competent to "fly solo." This orientation may range from 3 to 12 months, depending on the OR's specialty areas, a nurse's previous expertise, and a nurse's individual goals [2]. Didactic and clinical programs throughout the country also offer courses in perioperative nursing to individuals interested in pursuing this specialty area.

Throughout this issue, patient issues are discussed in some depth. Perioperative patient assessment and intervention are addressed and detail key issues. In her article on perioperative patient assessment, Ms. Bray points out "that patient education, and meeting the patient's spiritual, as well as physiological needs, demonstrates improved patient outcomes [7]. This has also led the way on how perioperative nurses conduct their pre-operative interview and assessment, and has tremendously improved the patient's recovery."

Complications that may develop intra- and postoperatively are discussed thoroughly by Ms. Wadlund. She indicates that the best tools available to the perioperative team are recognition and prevention [8]. Some postoperative complications are a result of patient positioning while under the influence of anesthesia. The importance of proper positioning techniques and the use of protective devices are covered fully in the article by Ms. O'Connell. She emphasizes the effects of anesthesia on patient receptors and subsequent response to pain, pressure, and positioning [9].

Laser and laparoscopic surgeries are explored in some detail. They pose specific risks in the surgical arena and are topics that may not be well understood by nurses outside the perioperative environment. In her article on laser surgery, Ms. Houck goes into detail about laser biophysics, laser safety, and surgical laser interventions [10]. In her article on laparoscopic interventions, Ms. Wadlund discusses the benefits, risks, and techniques of laparoscopy and the importance of having perioperative care plans in place for any circumstance that might arise [11].

Patients of every cultural, ethnic, and religious background are seen in the OR, and Ms. Quinn presents a thought-provoking article on the issues involved. The article stresses the importance of—and presents the need for—an understanding of patients, their ethnicity and cultural-religious values, and their personal history [14].

Morbidly obese patients recently have been a focus of much attention in the media. It has been an issue for perioperative nurses since the beginning, suddenly there has been an increased emphasis. Bariatric centers for the treatment of morbid obesity are springing up all over the country, which mandates serious discussion of the risks and benefits. Ms. Owens treats the topic with great sensitivity and understanding. She presents alarming statistics that affect patients of all ages [12,13].

Topics surrounding pediatric patients, pregnant patients, and geriatric patients also receive focus. The special needs and risks involved with these groups are given extensive review. In her article on pediatric patients, Ms. Ireland states the importance of remembering that they are not "miniature adults" (although the goals and standards of care remain the same as for adults). She presents the Erickson theory of personality development and how it impacts perioperative nursing care [15].

In Ms. Romanoski's article, which deals with pregnant surgical patients, issues often not well understood by perioperative nurses and nurses in general are brought to light. Being a cross-over specialty dictates the involvement of one or more specialties during surgical intervention [16]. Finally, a high percentage of surgical procedures are performed on geriatric patients. Ms. Mamaril delineates issues unique to this population in her discussion. Paramount to their care is treating the older population with understanding and respect, always remembering that age does not equate to intelligence—or lack thereof—and that elder patients were once young and productive [17].

SUMMARY

Everything that perioperative nurses do is patient focused, from the preoperative interview stage through postoperative discharge [18]. Perioperative nurses have the opportunity to share a subjective connection with patients while delivering care objectively [19]. It is necessary to have technical skills to obtain a satisfactory surgical outcome, which means that perioperative nurses must have a diverse knowledge of all surgical procedures. It is also essential to understand medications and their effects, the damaging effects of improper positioning, and how existing comorbidities can alter the surgical course. They also must know how to be astute observers and patient advocates.

In the words of the first perioperative nurse, Florence Nightingale, "It is quite incalculable the good that would certainly come from such sound and close observation in this almost neglected branch of nursing, or the help it would give to the medical man" [20].

Acknowledgments

I would like to extend my appreciation to Jane Rothrock, DNSc, JoAnne Connor, CRNFA, Maria Lorusso, and Jamie Horn for their invaluable suggestions.

Ms. Romanoski expresses her thanks to the following Paoli Hospital physicians for sharing their surgical, anesthesia and obstetrical expertise: Alex Anthopoulos, MD, James R. Bollinger, MD, David Robinson, MD, and Mojdeh Saberin-Williams, MD.

Gratia M. Nagle, RN, BA, CNOR, CRNFA, CRLS, CURN
5 Maude Circle
Paoli, PA 19301

E-mail address: GratiaNagle@cs.com

References

[1] Anonymous. Perioperative nursing. Available at: http://victorianfortunecity.com/rubens/386/ornursing.html. Accessed February 4, 2006.
[2] Fairchild SS. Now is the time/future of perioperative nursing. Available at: http://216.109.125.130/search/cache?p=Fairchild+%3A+now+is+the+future+of+perioperative+nursing&btn=Yahoo%21+Search&tab=Web&ei=UTF-8&u=southflorida.sun-sentinel.com/

careers/vitalsigns/pfold2001/xi22nowtim.htm&w=fairchild+now+future+perioperative+
nursing&d=Jd6gw21aMObc&icp=1&.intl=us. Accessed February 5, 2006.

[3] AORN. Standards, recommended practices, and guidelines. Denver (CO): AORN; 2005.

[4] Vaiden RE. Core curriculum for the RN first assistant. 4th edition. Denver (CO): AORN;
2005.

[5] Rothrock JC. Perioperative nursing care planning. 2nd edition. St. Louis (MO): Mosby;
1996.

[6] Phillips NF. Foundations of perioperative patient care standards. In: Berry and Kohn's operating room technique. 10th edition. St. Louis (MO): Mosby; 2004. p. 14.

[7] Oermann MH, Harris CH, Dammeyer JA. Teaching by the nurse: how important is it to patients? Appl Nurs Res 2001;14(1):11–7.

[8] Phillips NF. Potential preoperative complications. In: Berry and Kohn's operating room technique. 10th edition. St. Louis (MO): Mosby; 2004. p. 588–619.

[9] Guyton AC, Hall JE, editors. Textbook of medical physiology. 10th edition. Philadelphia (PA):
WB Saunders; 2000.

[10] Andersen K. Safe use of lasers in the operating room: what perioperative nurses should
know. AORN J 2004;79:171–88.

[11] Rothrock JC. Alexander's care of the patient in surgery. 12th edition. St. Louis (MO): Mosby;
2003.

[12] Flegal KM, Carroll MD, Ogden CL, et al. Prevalence and trends in obesity among US adults,
1999–2000. JAMA 2002;288:1723–7.

[13] Ogden CL, Flegal KM, Carroll MD, et al. Prevalence and trends in overweight among US
children and adolescents, 1999–2000. JAMA 2002;288:1728–32.

[14] Giger JN, Davidhizar RE. Transcultural nursing: assessment and intervention. 4th edition. St.
Louis (MO): Elsevier; 2004.

[15] Hockenberry MJ, Wilson D, Winkelstein ML, et al. Wong's nursing care of infants and children. 7th edition. St Louis (MO): Elsevier; 2003.

[16] Melnick DM, Wahl WL, Dalton VK. Management of general surgical problems in the pregnant patient. Am J Surg 2004;187(2):170–80.

[17] Anderson MA. Caring for older adults holistically. 3rd edition. Philadelphia (PA): FA Davis;
2003.

[18] Spry C. Essentials of perioperative nursing. 3rd edition. Sudbury (MA): Jones & Bartlett;
2005.

[19] Paulson DS. Taking care of patients and caring for patients are not the same. AORN J
2004;79(2):359–65.

[20] Nightingale F. Notes on nursing: what it is and what it is not. London: Harrison & Sons;
1859.

Nurs Clin N Am 41 (2006) 135–150

NURSING CLINICS
OF NORTH AMERICA

Preoperative Nursing Assessment of the Surgical Patient

Andrea Bray, RN, MSN, CNOR, RNFA

Highlands Ranch, CO, USA

Thorough assessment of the surgical patient begins in the preoperative phase and extends throughout the perioperative experience. Patient-centered interviews gather critical data that contribute to a successful experience and a focused plan of care. Information collected, documented, and conveyed to the surgeon or physician assists in appropriate medical decision making [1]. This article focuses on perioperative nursing assessment tools and discusses issues pertinent to achieving safe delivery of care. A broad overview touches on key topics that deserve exploration and evaluation. This article will hopefully serve as a useful tool that helps direct the decision-making process.

Long before the existence of operating room suites, physicians performed surgical procedures on kitchen tables, battlefields, and barber chairs. Nurses who assisted the surgeon were sent to the patient's home to prepare a suitable area for the procedure. In the nineteenth century as advancements in technology evolved, concern for patient safety and the cleanliness of the surgical area increased. Hospitals began building operating suites and improving methods of asepsis. During the early 1920s, just as now, nurses were the primary advocates for the surgical patient. Research studies during the 1960s and 1970s showed a correlation between preoperative assessment, patient preparation, and postoperative outcomes [2]. Research shows that patient outcomes improve with patient education and when the patient's spiritual and physiologic needs are met [3]. This finding has been instrumental in the development of preoperative interview and assessment tools for perioperative nurses, and has tremendously improved patient recovery.

In 2002, the American Society of Anesthesiologists (ASA) Task Force on Preanesthesia Evaluation released a practice advisory report [4]. This tool helps direct decision making in patient care when no scientific evidence exists.

E-mail address: bray36@comcast.net

PRELIMINARY ASSESSMENT

Determining how well the patient understands the intended surgical procedure gives the perioperative nurse an idea of how much support the patient will receive from their family for such things as coughing and deep breathing, encouraging ambulation, and pain control [5]. Family support has become essential over the past decade with the increased numbers of procedures performed in physicians' offices, free-standing ambulatory surgicenters, and hospital-based surgicenter [6].

The increasing number of surgeries performed outside of the traditional hospital operating room has prompted a different preoperative assessment because the patient is no longer "worked up" in the conventional manner with EKGs, laboratory studies, and chest radiographs. The perioperative nurse in these alternative settings must carefully assess the patient to a level that is comfortable for both patient and nurse and allows a safe advancement of surgical progression [7]. Vital information for the nurse to obtain includes, but is not limited to, height, weight, allergies, comorbidities, and current medications. Identifying the specific types of allergies is a key component in providing a safe environment. If the patient has a latex allergy, for example, some supplies such as tubing and gloves may need to be replaced with latex-free items. Many operating rooms have converted to essentially latex-free environments for this reason.

The goals of the preoperative assessment are to assemble information with the patient and establish an intraoperative plan of care while respecting the patient's individual goals and preferences [8]. Research has shown that this assessment and planning have decreased the morbidity and mortality of the patient during the perioperative period. Communication between the perioperative nurse and the preoperative surgical patient improves recovery and helps prevent problems in the operating room [9]. Collaboration with the patient better enables the perioperative nurse to obtain information necessary for appropriate diagnosis, planning, and implementation of care [10].

Physical examination of the patient is also crucial because it enables the nurse to visualize any abnormal findings, ask the patient about these findings, and document the findings in the preoperative record [11]. The assessment performed by the perioperative nurse helps guide the care given to each individual patient throughout the perioperative experience [1]. The assessment also allows the perioperative nurse to make accurate nursing diagnoses, identify the educational needs of the patient and family, and implement the interventions necessary to achieve desired outcomes [12].

Recently, the trend has been to move surgical procedures from the hospital to physician's offices; facilities attached and adjacent to the hospital; and freestanding ambulatory centers. In today's shortened hospital stay, the patient may arrive at the surgical facility only 1 to 2 hours before the scheduled surgery. The preoperative assessment becomes a crucial element in intervention, outcome planning, patient education, and planning for discharge to ensure the patient's safety and desired outcome [13].

Thorough patient assessment by the perioperative nurse will help determine if the patient is an appropriate candidate to undergo a surgical procedure at a physician's office, a free-standing surgicenter, the main operating suite, or the hospital-based surgicenter [4,14]. After speaking with the patient and obtaining their past medical and surgical history, the nurse must determine if any other tests would help create the best possible outcome for that patient [15]. Other factors that may influence the choice of surgical setting is the patient's mental status and age [16]. A younger patient who is of sound mind would be a more appropriate candidate to undergo surgery in the surgicenter setting than a person who has dementia [17].

The amount and type of rehabilitation services needed after the procedure also influence the appropriateness of the facility. A patient requiring extensive physical or occupational therapy may not be a good candidate for the surgicenter unless they reside in a nursing home where this therapy can be ordered after they return. Another factor to consider is the likelihood of a blood transfusion. Any medical conditions that keep the patient from clotting appropriately should be examined closely before a decision is made as to which facility is most appropriate [18]. The presence of family support and trust is instrumental in determining if the patient will receive the help and support they need after surgery and who they can contact if they need additional support [4,6,7,18]. Cost-effectiveness is also something to consider when determining which facility is most appropriate.

Thorough assessment imparts a sense of trust and care from the perioperative nurse to the patient. A patient assessment form (Fig. 1) given to the patient before the interview helps provide the operating team better insight into the patient's history. An assessment form completed by the patient, or family member if the patient is unable, helps the perioperative nurse identify any areas of concern and explore the situation further. These assessment forms help the perioperative nurse complete a timely and organized evaluation of the patient.

COMMUNICATION

When speaking with the patient for the first time in the preoperative holding area, perioperative nurses should introduce themselves to the patient and family using a strong, understandable tone of voice. The name tag should be visible and available for the patient to view [19]. Surgical masks should not be worn and eye contact should be made with the patient and family. The perioperative nurse should acknowledge the questions and concerns of the family and patient.

Groundwork for a satisfactory experience involves establishing a relationship with the patient; becoming familiar with and gaining specific information about the medical history and symptom profile; having a knowledge base of the impending surgical procedure; and determining family support [4,15]. If the patient's family is not physically present during the preoperative interview, the perioperative nurse should determine how to contact them once the procedure is finished.

Saint Joseph's Hospital of Atlanta
ADMISSION ASSESSMENT

PART 1: COMPLETED BY PATIENT

▸ = Enter these items in MIS computer
▸ Unable to answer questions due to:_____

I. SPECIAL NEEDS   ☐ None known

▸ 1. Allergies (Medications, food, other)
     List   Reaction
     _____   _____
     _____   _____
     _____   _____
     _____   _____

▸ 2. Previous blood transfusions   ☐ Yes ☐ No
     If yes, when (date)_____

     Reactions (Problems):   ☐ Yes ☐ No
     Describe_____
▸ 3. Have you given blood for your use? ☐ Yes ☐ No
▸ 4. Has anyone donated blood for your use? ☐ Yes ☐ No
  5. Have you been exposed to measles, mumps
     or chicken pox in last 3 weeks?   ☐ Yes ☐ No
  6. If you are female, are you:
         Pregnant   ☐ Yes ☐ No
         Having your period   ☐ Yes ☐ No
         Wearing a tampon   ☐ Yes ☐ No
▸ 7. Do you have any limitations in following areas: ☐ No
         ☐ Hearing   Describe_____
     _____

         ☐ Eyesight   Describe_____
     _____

         ☐ Language Barrier Describe_____
     _____

Past Hospitalizations / Surgeries:_____
_____
_____

Have you ever been a patient at Saint Joseph's Hospital?
☐ No   ☐ Yes When_____
_____

Saint Joseph's Hospital of Atlanta
ADMISSION ASSESSMENT
Approved by MRC: 6/92

II. MEDICAL PROBLEMS / PAST HOSPITALIZATION:

	Past	Current
1. Lung Disease	☐	☐
2. Shortness of breath	☐	☐
3. Asthma	☐	☐
4. Emphyscma	☐	☐
5. Tuberculosis	☐	☐
6. Chronic cough	☐	☐
7. Abnormal Chest X-ray	☐	☐
8. Heart Disease	☐	☐
9. Chest Pain / Angina	☐	☐
10. Heart Attack	☐	☐
11. Hypertension (high blood pressure)	☐	☐
12. Hypotension (low blood pressure)	☐	☐
13. Pacemaker	☐	☐
14. Abnormal EKG	☐	☐
15. Stroke (CVA)	☐	☐
16. Muscle Weakness / Disease	☐	☐
17. Back/Neck problems	☐	☐
18. Arthritis	☐	☐
19. Broken bones	☐	☐
20. Epilepsy	☐	☐
21. Dizziness	☐	☐
22. Migraines	☐	☐
23. Confusion	☐	☐
24. Blackouts	☐	☐
25. Motion sickness	☐	☐
26. Diabetes	☐	☐
27. Hypoglycemia (low blood sugar)	☐	☐
28. Nose Surgery	☐	☐
29. Thyroid or goiter	☐	☐
30. Bleeding or clotting disorder	☐	☐
31. Anemia	☐	☐
32. Cancer	☐	☐
33. Tumors	☐	☐
34. Prostate Disease	☐	☐
35. Stomach / Bowel Problems	☐	☐
36. Kidney / Bladder Problems	☐	☐
37. Liver Disease	☐	☐
38. Hepatitis (yellow jaundice)	☐	☐
39. Chronic Pain	☐	☐
40. Skin condition	☐	☐
41. Carrier of contagious disease	☐	☐
42. Glaucoma	☐	☐

Other Medical Problems / Comments:_____
_____

(Part 1 continued on next page)

NAME_____

Fig. 1. Sample of perioperative patient assessment form. (A) Predesigned admission assessment form in a check-off format brought with the patient from the physician's office can speed up the admission process. (B) Assessment data provides information to formulate nursing diagnoses and plan interventions. (Courtesy of St. Joseph's Hospital of Atlanta.)

Successful communication with the patient can be achieved through patient-centered behavior that enhances the patient's personal integrity and value. Whatever the circumstances, nurses who are nonjudgmental and provide a caring atmosphere make the patient feel comfortable and instill a feeling of well-being, making patients feel as though they really matter after all. Qualities that display this to a patient include being attentive, connected, friendly,

► = Enter these items in MIS computer.

PART 2: COMPLETED BY HOSPITAL PERSONNEL

DISCHARGE PLANNING / EDUCATION / PSYCHOSOCIAL ASSESSMENT

. □ Pre-op Teaching _____ R.N.

. Areas which may require patient teaching and/or assistance prior to discharge:
- □ Pre-op teaching
- □ Medications
- □ Prep for DX procedures
- □ Wound Care
- □ Dietary instructions
- □ Food preparation
- □ Social Service Consult / Discharge Planning
- □ Integumentary
- □ Self Care _____
- □ Diabetic reactions
- □ Cardiac rehabilitation
- □ Mobility
- □ Physical layout of home
- □ Transportation

□ Post Procedure needs_____

□ Other educational needs_____

I. ADMISSION DATA

1. Date_____
2. Time_____
3. NPO since _____
4. Accompanied to hospital by_____
5. Are you wearing □ false eyelashes □ wig/hairpiece

    □ other prostheses Specify:_____
6. Armband on: □ Yes □ No
7. Special needs armband on & chart labeled: □ Yes □ No
8. Admitted to Room_____ from

    □ Home   □ Nursing Home

    □ Another Hospital_____

    □ Other_____
9. Treated in: □ ED □ ERC □ Cath Lab

    □ Other_____
10. Information obtained from_____

Saint Joseph's Hospital of Atlanta
ADMISSION ASSESSMENT
Approved by MRC: 6/92

III. VITAL STATISTICS

1. Temperature_____ □ Ax/Tym. □ Oral □ Rectal
2. Pulse_____
3. Respirations_____
4. Blood Pressure _____ Right Arm _____ Left Arm
5. □ Right handed or □ Left handed
► 6. Height_____
► 7. Weight_____
    □ Standing scale   □ Bedscale   □ Chair scale

IV. SAFETY / WELL-BEING

Patient/Family oriented to:	Restricted	Yes	No
1. Primary Care Delivery Model		□	□
2. Bed operation	□	□	□
3. Call Bell		□	□
4. Bathroom	□	□	□
5. Bathroom emergency call light	□	□	□
6. Visiting Policy	□	□	□
7. Television	□	□	□
8. Meal times	□	□	□
9. Telephone	□	□	□
10. Siderails		□	□
11. Name on door		□	□
12. Face Sheet signed by patient/authorized person		□	□
13. Advanced Directives Checklist on chart & signed		□	□
14. Valuables policy		□	□
15. Disposal of valuables/medications_____			

Additional comments_____

Fig. 1 (continued)

helpful, unobtrusive, and respectful [20], especially when dealing with younger and older patients [16,18,20].

INTERVENTION

Depending on the procedure, patients who have hearing aids may be allowed to wear them during surgery. The perioperative nurse needs to ask the patient how to adjust the hearing device if it starts to malfunction during the procedure. Often patients may wear their glasses into the operating suite if they choose. If the glasses are removed intraoperatively they should be labeled and placed in a secure location. The glasses will be returned in the recovery room. Contact lenses should be removed before the patient leaves the preoperative area because they can dry out and scratch the patient's cornea.

For patients who are blind, additional interventions may be necessary to make them feel secure. Nurses should always speak before making any physical contact and should remember that the patient is blind and not deaf; speaking in a normal yet audible tone is preferable to raising one's voice or shouting. The perioperative nurse should verbally describe what is going on in the surroundings and warn of unexpected noises, if possible.

The anesthesiologist should decide if the patient is allowed to wear dentures during surgery. Retained dentures can often help in airway maintenance and the safer induction of anesthesia. A better seal between the oxygen mask and mouth can be achieved when dentures are worn. If the patient has a prosthetic device, the perioperative nurse and anesthesiologist should decide together if the patient may wear the prosthetic into the operating suite, and if not, the device should be properly contained and identified with a patient label. It may be placed under the patient gurney or removed and stored in the hospital room if the patient has been admitted.

DATA COLLECTION

The chart should contain the patient's medical history and should be reviewed with the patient at the beginning of the interview. The patient history will help the perioperative nurse and medical team determine the most appropriate diagnoses and care. When reviewing the medical history, the nurse should inquire about prior hospitalizations and outcomes because preexisting diseases can alter the implementation of patient care and the surgical outcome. Having a perioperative nurse who is knowledgeable of the medical history is often reassuring for patients who are feeling anxious. Delving beyond the obvious is important in constructing the framework for nursing diagnoses [1,15].

Obtaining the patient's anesthetic and surgical history is also important. This information allows the perioperative team to better prepare and anticipate the patient's needs and prevent any complications from arising, such as malignant hyperthermia. The perioperative nurse must also check the chart to see that a history and physical have been completed and dated within the hospital protocol time frame. The surgical and anesthesia consent forms must also be in the chart, signed by the provider and the patient.

LEGAL ISSUES

If the patient has a medical power of attorney, living will, or advance directive, copies should be placed in the chart where they are easily accessible. If the advance directive indicates that the patient has chosen not to be resuscitated, the request is commonly terminated during surgery. Many hospitals have begun to implement an additional form that allows the patient to decide what measures they would like performed in the operating room. The anesthesiologist, surgeon, and perioperative nurse are all allowed to express their opinions and discuss the various ethical issues and implications of advance directives with the patient.

The Association of Operating Room Nurses (AORN) position statement on the perioperative care of patients who have do not resuscitate (DNR) orders states that the surgical team must respect the patient's autonomy and is responsible for documenting the information provided [8]. This documentation should include the purpose of the operation, the likelihood of resuscitative measures, a detailed explanation of what resuscitative measures are included, and what the potential outcomes may be with and without resuscitation. If the patient chooses to suspend their DNR order during surgery, when the DNR will be reinstated must be documented. If for any reason the perioperative nurse is uncomfortable with the patient's decisions, they have the right to request that another nurse assume the patient's care. If another nurse is not available, the patient's wishes take precedence.

The perioperative nurse may eventually face a difficult ethical dilemma, such as providing care for a patient who is unresponsive and whose family has not been notified of the injuries. The perioperative nurse's role is to act as the patient's advocate and intervene with appropriate choices and solutions. Situations may arise in the operating room when the behavior of the surgeon is questionable or an error in technique or procedure occurs with the demand that no documentation be made. Times such as these can become emotionally difficult for the perioperative nurse, but the responsibility of protecting the patient requires a response in accordance with the professional codes of conduct [21]. These codes of conduct for perioperative nurses include (1) accountability for actions and expectations, and (2) responsibility to the public, health care team, and nursing profession.

Failure to comply with these standards may result in dismissal, suspension, or loss of nursing license. If perioperative nurses ever have a question or believe they are being put in a difficult position, they should contact the facility's ethics committee or the state board of nursing. One role of the ethics committee is to providing perioperative nurses with the tools to address such situations. The ethics committee can also provide guidance with advance directives, DNR orders, living wills, medical power of attorney, patient concerns, patient rights, patient confidentiality, and protocols [21].

INTRAOPERATIVE RISKS

Patients should be asked open-ended questions to determine how well they complied with any preoperative orders given by the physician or anesthesiologist. The level of compliance can influence the type of anesthesia used. This information may include whether or not the patient followed the NPO orders or discontinued the use of anticoagulants in an appropriate time frame. If the patient is at risk for aspiration, cricoid pressure may be needed or a regional anesthetic may be considered. Current NPO guidelines state that patients should not have eaten within 8 hours before surgery, although an exception is made in emergent surgery and clear liquids can be consumed up until 2 to

3 hours preoperatively. Physicians may encourage patients to take all oral medications with a small sip of water on the day of their procedure. The surgeon or anesthesiologist may give special instructions for small children, patients who have diabetes, and elderly patients who may be prone to dehydration [4,14]. The ASA has established guidelines for the perioperative nurse regarding the preoperative administration of insulin therapy (Fig. 2) [4].

During the preoperative assessment, the nurse should ensure that the patient has removed all jewelry, including belly button rings and other piercings. This issue should be addressed specifically, with explanations of the potential

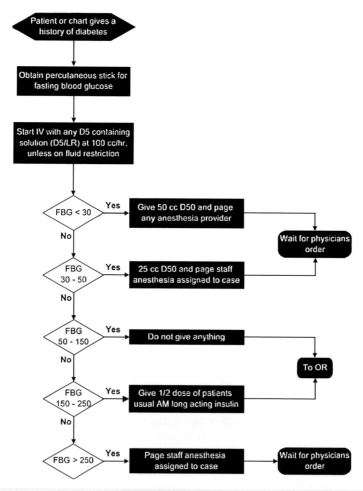

Fig. 2. Algorithm for patient who has diabetes. AM, morning; FBG, fasting blood glucose; IV, intravenous line; OR, operating room (*From* Maurer WG, Borkowski RG, Parker BM. Quality and resource utilization in managing preoperative evaluation. Anesthesiol Clin North America 2004;22:164; with permission.)

hazards. Many patients forget or neglect to inform the perioperative nurse of body piercings, and therefore the perioperative nurse must ask specifically has about any body piercings and explain that their removal is important in preventing burns from the electrocautery [22]. All patients should be asked about body piercings regardless of age.

MEDICAL HISTORY

Assessment of the surgical patient should also include information such as the patient's general health status, skin condition, mobility restrictions, and prescription medications or over-the-counter products the patient may be using. Any antihypertensive, antianginal, antiarrhythmic, anticoagulation, anticonvulsant, and diabetic medications should be noted [4]. Some of these medications can adversely affect anesthetic agents or may impact the physiologic response and hemodynamic outcome of the surgical procedure [23].

For patients who have insulin-dependent diabetes, the multiorgan nature of the disease and patient assessment measures must be addressed. The ASA developed a nursing algorithm for diabetes mellitus to guide insulin administration in the preoperative arena (see Fig. 2). This algorithm provides guidance on timing of drug administration, notifying the anesthesia team, and delaying transfer of the patient to the operating room [4].

Identifying any illicit drug use, cigarette smoking, and alcohol consumption is important because these influence the patient's anesthetic tolerance, increase nausea and vomiting, and may cause the patient to experience a malignant hyperthermia crisis. Nicotine withdrawal may cause the patient to become irritable and anxious. The amount of alcohol the patient consumes may also increase the patient's tolerance to anesthesia, requiring more than normal amounts of anesthesia to be administered. Postoperatively, the perianesthesia nurse must be aware of peripheral neuropathy after the use of regional anesthetics [24].

RISKS FOR POSITIONAL INJURY

Any specific areas of potential skin breakdown on the patient's extremities should be identified to help with patient positioning and lessen the discomfort. Because the skin is the body's first line of defense against foreign bodies, the perioperative nurse must assess and identify breaks in the patient's skin that may increase the risk for infection [25].

Elderly patients must be examined closely for any areas of skin breakdown or pressure points. The elderly patient's skin tends to be very thin and fragile, making them more susceptible to positional pressure-point injury during surgery.

Patients who are obese and in the supine position often desaturate quickly. Therefore, the perioperative nurse may want to use the semi-Fowler position when taking the patient to and from the operating suite and use a pillow or other positioning device on the operative bed to elevate the patient's head. Patients who are obese also have a higher gastric content and lower pH. Cricoid pressure should be used on induction to help prevent the risk for aspiration. When assessing these patients, the perioperative nurse must ensure that the operating bed can support the patient's weight. The manufacturer's instructions or sales representative can help determine the table's allowable weight limit. Additional positioning devices, such as a toboggan, may be necessary to accommodate the patient's size. In some instances, two tables have been strapped together to accommodate patients who are morbidly obese.

Patients who have arthritis, contractures, or other physical impairments have an inherently increased risk for developing pressure sores. Additional and inventive padding or positioning may be required to prevent complications. After assessing the patient and evaluating the body habitus and physical limitations, the perioperative nurse should plan ahead and gather additional personnel to assist with moving the patient. Proper assessment, planning, and implementation will assist in alleviating many untoward events [2,12].

In the past, sequential circulating devices (SCDs) were only worn by patients who presented with a high risk for developing an embolism. Currently, however, most surgical patients are being required to wear the SCDs during the operation as a preventative measure to guard against thrombophlebitis and a thromboembolism. When assessing the patient, the perioperative nurse should ensure that these SCDs and their machine either have been applied to the patient's lower extremities or are available on the patient's gurney.

Care must be taken when asking the patient about allergies. What type of allergic reaction occurs if the patient encounters an allergen is important to note. True allergic reactions include pruritus with hives or flushing; facial or oral swelling; difficulty breathing or shortness of breath; choking; wheezing; or vascular collapse. Allergies to seafood or shellfish may cause a reaction when intravenous contrast dye, certain preparatory solutions, and some anesthetic medications such as protamine are used. All allergies must be verified with the patient (or family if the patient is unable to communicate), documented on the front of the patients chart, and identified on the patient's wristband. Identifying if any blood relatives have had difficulty with anesthesia or have a known allergy to succinylcholine is beneficial to reducing the patient's chance of experiencing a malignant hyperthermia crisis.

Determining if the patient has sensitive skin may help the perioperative nurse decide which antimicrobial agent to use for skin preparation and whether to use a povidone-iodine, alcohol, or chlorhexidine gluconate preparation, or baby shampoo. If the patient has sensitive skin and the surgeon prefers one antimicrobial agent, such as Betadine and alcohol, the perioperative nurse should inform the surgeon of the patient's potential problem and suggest a more suitable alternative.

EDUCATION

Patient education is crucial for the patient and family. With shorter hospital stays, care is the responsibility of the patient and their family. Educational pamphlets provide written instructions that augment what is conveyed verbally and repeat specific information (Fig. 3). Although most material is written at a third grade reading level, the perioperative nurse must ascertain that the patient is able to read and comprehend the written material. Written instructions also help clarify any misunderstood or forgotten information once the patient is home. Patients who do not speak English must be given special consideration [26]. Many companies prepare pamphlets in Spanish. If another language is spoken, the facility must provide an interpreter and a contact list should be available. Consideration must be given to patients from cultural backgrounds who find it inappropriate for a man to interpret (or care) for a woman and vise-versa. Other cultures require a family elder to be present when making any decisions.

As the perioperative nurse develops a relationship with the patient, additional educational needs of the patient and family can be discovered, evaluated, and managed. Important information includes the patient's understanding of the impending procedure. This understanding helps build the framework of the objectives and outcomes for the patient. If the patient's anxiety level is

PREOPERATIVE INSTRUCTIONS

Your doctor has scheduled your surgery to be performed at Getbetter Hospital on _____ (date) _____ at _____ AM/PM. Please arrive at _____ AM/PM.

If you develop a cold, flu, or illness before surgery or cannot keep your surgery appointment, please call your surgeon.

DIETARY RESTRICTIONS
- Avoid alcoholic beverages and cigarette smoking for at least 24 hours before surgery.
- Finish dinner the evening before surgery no later than 8 PM.
- Nothing to eat or drink after midnight the night before surgery.
  (This includes candy, gum, mints, Lifesavers, ice chips, and water.)
- Eating or drinking may result in the delay or cancellation of surgery.
- Medications to be taken the day of surgery _____ with sip (1 ounce) of water.
- Medications not to be taken the day of surgery _____ .

FOR YOUR SAFETY AND COMFORT
- No makeup—it may cause eye irritation or corneal abrasions while under anesthesia.
- Remove nail polish and artificial nails from at least one finger on each hand—oxygen is measured by placing a sensor on your finger tip.
- Do not bring valuables or jewelry—jewelry must be removed before surgery.
- Dress simply in loose-fitting clothes (sweatsuits are ideal).

UPON YOUR ARRIVAL
- Report to Main Lobby Admissions Desk.

AFTER YOUR SURGERY
- No driving, operating of heavy machinery, heavy physical activity, or decision making for 24 hours after receiving an anesthetic.
- If you are returning home on the same day as your surgery, make arrangements for a responsible adult to accompany you. Your operation cannot be performed if a responsible adult is not with you.
- Call your surgeon for postoperative appointments.

If you have any questions, do not hesitate to call the Preadmission Testing Unit at xxx-xxx-xxxx or The Department of Anesthesia at xxx-xxx-xxxx.

Patient signature: _____

RN signature: _____

Fig. 3. Patient preoperative instruction form. (*From* Phillips N. Berry & Kohn's operating room technique. 10th edition. St. Louis (MO): Mosby; 2004. p. 366; with permission.)

high, identifying the sources of the anxiety and providing reassurance and support may help alleviate some of the anxiety. An patient who is anxious will not be able to concentrate or comprehend information provided by the perioperative nurse.

Many anxieties stem from the patient's self-image; role status; medical and family expenses; knowledge deficit; and fear of dying. Signs that may indicate anxiety include

- Increased heart rate
- Increased or fluctuating blood pressure
- Rapid respiratory rate
- Trembling in the voice
- Fidgeting of hands
- Avoiding eye contact

Patients should be reassured that they will be accompanied by a member of the perioperative team at all times and they will not ever be left alone for any reason. This practice can help establish a sense of trust and security for the patient and family. Asking open-ended questions and allowing patients to express their biggest concerns in a nonjudgmental environment are the easiest ways to establish an appropriate teaching plan for individual patients and their family. Once the concerns are addressed, anxiety levels decrease. Determining the amount of family support the patient will have after discharge can help reassure the patient. If no family support is available, the perioperative nurse can help establish a plan for home health care or arrange support from a friend. Determining how well the patient comprehends the expected outcome can help the patient during postoperative recovery. The patient is likely to be more comfortable with the impending surgery if they know the expected outcome. The nurse should provide as much time as necessary to explain the details of what is and will be occurring. Recognizing and respecting how much detail the patient wants to know helps the patient feel comfortable.

The nurse should offer matter-of-fact information and not elaborate descriptions. The patient's desire and ability to acquire more information should be assessed and that information should be provided as appropriate. The patient should be informed of where they will go after the procedure and what they can expect postoperatively. The patient should be encouraged to ask for postoperative assistance, and any other pertinent precautions that are specific to the patient and type of surgery should be related. For example, a patient undergoing a total hip arthroplasty must ask for assistance before getting out of bed. The nurse should remember to speak in a calm, slow voice and take as much time as needed to educate the patient and family of essential information. Too much information too fast can be overwhelming. Using medical terminology may confuse the patient. If tests are ordered, such as an EKG, the nurse can help reassure the patient and alleviate fears by explaining why. Assisting the family with directions to the waiting area and where they can find food and drinks can help to minimize their anxiety.

Patients may have concerns about pain after their procedure. An estimated 30 million patients per year experience uncontrolled postoperative pain. Once the patient's tissue has been traumatized from surgery, the pain receptors send a message to the spinal column, which excites chemical mediators. These chemical mediators then excite the nerve fibers at the operative site, increasing the level of pain. The Agency for Health Care Policy and Research claims that postoperative pain is typically caused by incommensurate medication.

The numeric pain scale is a straightforward way for patients to understand and indicate their status, thus allowing sufficient pain relief (Fig. 4). If a patient is unable to follow the numeric scale, other scales such as the facial expression scale (Fig. 5) may be easier to use. Explaining the pain scale to patients before surgery can help them control pain after the procedure. Using the pain scale to relate previous experiences to practice may be helpful for the patient. The perioperative nurse should communicate to the patient that it is the patient's responsibility to tell the staff when their pain begins to reach an intolerable level [27].

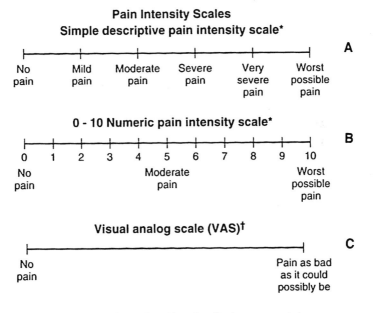

Pain Intensity Scales
Simple descriptive pain intensity scale*

A

No pain   Mild pain   Moderate pain   Severe pain   Very severe pain   Worst possible pain

0 - 10 Numeric pain intensity scale*

B

0 1 2 3 4 5 6 7 8 9 10
No pain   Moderate pain   Worst possible pain

Visual analog scale (VAS)†

C

No pain   Pain as bad as it could possibly be

* If used as a graphic rating scale, a 10-cm baseline is recommended.
† A 10-cm baseline is recommended for VAS scales.

Which face shows how much hurt you have now?

Fig. 4. (A-C) Numeric pain scale. (*From* Rothrock JC. Alexander's care of the patient in surgery. 12th edition. St. Louis (MO): Mosby; 2003. p. 269; with permission.)

Which face shows how much hurt you have now?

0	1	2	3	4	5
No hurt	Hurts little bit	Hurts little more	Hurts even more	Hurts whole lot	Hurts worst

Fig. 5. Facial (FACES) pain scale rating. (*From* Hockenberry MJ, Wilson D, Winkelstein ML. Wong's essentials of pediatric nursing, 7th edition. St. Louis (MO): Mosby; 2005. p. 1259; with permission.)

Providing a realistic expectation of the postoperative pain can also help alleviate the patient's anxiety. The perioperative nurse should educate the patient before surgery on deep breathing exercises. The nurse should explain that deep breathing and ambulating as soon as possible, even though these practices may be uncomfortable, can accelerate recovery time and help alleviate pain faster. Other nonpharmacologic methods to reduce pain may include listening to music, aromatherapy, or the patient's choice of distraction methods [28]. Patients must be taught that the goal of pain management is to keep pain at a tolerable level, rather than to request medication when the pain becomes unbearable.

Medicating around-the-clock rather than on a PRN basis has been shown to be more effective in pain control. When administering around-the-clock medication, the nurse must ensure that the patient does not become oversedated. Pain medication may be given in combination with other medications, such as nonsteriodal anti-inflammatory drugs (NSAIDS) combined with opioids. Certain NSAIDs must be used with caution, however, because of their effect on coagulation and platelet activity. Providing preoperative education about these choices can help patients decide if their pain level might benefit from combining medication.

Patients may not fully comprehend preoperative explanations of what they might experience postoperatively. However, once they emerge from anesthesia, awareness of what is happening to them and why is often reassuring. Recovery time is dependent on the type of procedure. The perioperative nurse must explain that it often takes several months for patients to completely recover from procedures. The recovery process is often accelerated when the patient is educated to take it easy even when they feel terrific.

Discussing the signs and symptoms of infection and other information that would require patients to call their surgeon sooner than usual can not only help alleviate fear but also help them recover faster. Nurses should encourage patients to call the surgeon immediately with any questions they may have rather than to wait, because the surgeon may determine an urgent need to see the patient that could potentially save that patient's life or prevent a large, multisystem infection [25].

Establishing a communication plan with the family while the patient is in surgery can help alleviate the family's stress and anxiety. When the perioperative nurse and the family have agreed on a time of communication, the perioperative nurse must remember to call out to the family at that designated time. Some hospitals are implementing a registered-nurse liaison, who establishes a relationship with the family in the preoperative phase, then checks with the surgeon each hour and directly communicates with the family in the waiting area, giving them updates and answering questions. This concept has been favorably received by families and has greatly reduced their worry.

DISCHARGE PLANNING

Perioperative nurses are becoming more involved in the discharge planning because of the increasing number of procedures occurring in alternative same-day settings. Discharge planning starts with the preoperative assessment through identifying the patient's mental, physical, and psychosocial needs. Assessing the patient and family's understanding of the care that will be needed after discharge helps identify what services may be required. The perioperative nurse may collaborate with the case management, social services, physical and occupational therapy rehabilitative services, pastoral representatives, financial services, and home health care network [29]. Case management and social services should be advised immediately of any additional help the patient will require after discharge. Early notification can reduce the length of the hospital stay and help prevent readmission.

SUMMARY

Thorough and accurate patient assessment is vital to the patient's long-term outcome. The preoperative phase has become increasingly more important for accomplishing desired outcomes. At the end of the perioperative nurse's assessment, patients' anxiety levels should be decreased because of the education they received. To confirm the patient's understanding, the nurse might ask, "What problems may arise that would be important for you to call your physician?"

References

[1] Brannon LA, Carson KL. Nursing expertise and information structure influence medical decision making. Appl Nurs Res 2003;16(4):287–90.

[2] Phillips N. Berry & Kohn's operating room technique. 10th edition. St. Louis (MO): Mosby; 2004.

[3] Oermann MH, Harris CH, Dammeyer JA. Teaching by the nurse: how important is it to patients? Appl Nurs Res 2001;14(1):11–7

[4] Maurer WG, Borkowski RG, Parker BM. Quality and resource utilization in managing preoperative evaluation. Anesthesiol Clin North America 2004;22:155–75.

[5] Li H. Identifying family care process themes in caring for their hospitalized elders. Appl Nurs Res 2005;18(2):97–101.

[6] Majasaari H, Sarajarvi A, Koskinen H. Patients' perceptions of emotional support and information to family members. AORN J 2005;81(5):1030–8.

[7] DeLamar LM. Preparing your patient for surgery, topics in advanced practice nursing. Available at: www.medscape.com. Accessed December 2005.

[8] AORN. Standards, recommended practices, and guidelines. Denver (CO): The Association; 2005.

[9] Canobbio MM. Mosby's handbook of patient teaching. 3rd edition. St. Louis (MO): Elsevier; 2006.

[10] Hutchisson B, Phippen ML, Papanier-Wells M. Review of perioperative nursing. Philadelphia: Saunders; 2000.

[11] LeBlond RF, DeGowin RL, Brown DD. DeGowin's diagnostic examination. New York: McGraw-Hill; 2004.

[12] Rothrock JC. Alexander's care of the patient in surgery. 12th edition. St. Louis (MO): Mosby; 2003.

[13] London F. How to prepare families for discharge in the limited time available. Pediatr Nurs 2004;30(3):212–4, 227.

[14] Hurford WE, Bailn MT, Davison JK, et al. Clinical anesthesia procedures of the Massachusetts General Hospital. 6th edition. Philadelphia: Lippincott Williams & Wilkins; 2002.

[15] Brannon LA, Carson KL. The representativeness heuristic: influence on nurses' decision making. Appl Nurs Res 2003;16(3):201–4.

[16] Saufl NM. Preparing the older adult for surgery and anesthesia. J Perianesth Nurs 2004;19(6):372–8.

[17] Wakefield BJ. Behaviors and outcomes of acute confusion in hospitalized patients. Appl Nurs Res 2002;14(4):209–16.

[18] Busen NH. Perioperative preparation of the adolescent surgical patient. AORN J 2001;73(2):37–62.

[19] Lange JW. Patient identification of caregivers' title: do they know who you are? Appl Nurs Res 2002;15(1):11–8

[20] Jacelon CS. Attitudes and behaviors of hospital staff toward elders in an acute care setting. Appl Nurs Res 2002;15(4):227–34.

[21] Brownsey D. Nurses and their right to whistle blow. AORN J 2001;73(3):693–7. (www.whistleblowers.org/private.htm)

[22] Larkin BG. The ins and outs of body piercings. AORN J 2004;79(2):333–42.

[23] Miller CA. Safe medication practices: nursing assessment of medications in older adults. Geriatr Nurs 2003;24(5):314–5, 317.

[24] DeFazio-Quinn DM, Schick L. Perianesthesia nursing core curriculum. Philadelphia: Saunders; 2004.

[25] Gruendemann BJ, Mangum SS. Infection prevention in surgical settings. Philadelphia: Saunders; 2001.

[26] Dreger V, Trembeck T. Optimize patient health by treating literacy and language barriers. AORN J 2002;75(2):279–93.

[27] Heye ML, Foster L, Bartlett MK, et al. A preoperative intervention for pain reduction, improved mobility, and self-efficacy. Appl Nurs Res 2002;15(3):174–83.

[28] Smolen D, Tropp R, Singer L. The effect of self-selected music during colonoscopy on anxiety, heart rate, and blood pressure. Appl Nurs Res 2002;16(2):126–36.

[29] Bowles KH, Foust JB, Naylor MD. Hospital discharge referral decision making: a multidisciplinary perspective. Appl Nurs Res 2003;16(3):134–43.

Nurs Clin N Am 41 (2006) 151–171

NURSING CLINICS
OF NORTH AMERICA

ELSEVIER
SAUNDERS

Prevention, Recognition, and Management of Nursing Complications in the Intraoperative and Postoperative Surgical Patient

Diana L. Wadlund, RN, CRNFA, CRNP

Surgical Specialists, 1351 Julieanna Drive, West Chester, PA 19380, USA

P erioperative complications are unexpected, potentially devastating events that have serious consequences for not only the surgical patient but also the team of health care providers that care for him or her. Postoperative complications delay the patient's return to normal life and function. Additionally, they potentially can cause the death of the patient and give the surgical team a feeling of failure even when there clearly was no way to avoid the complication [1].

In reviewing the literature, the one thing that stood out most acutely was that the best way to deal with complications was to simply prevent them from happening. Highlighted time and again was the need for accurate, thorough preoperative assessment of the surgical patient. This helps to identify potential risks for surgical complications and to allow the surgical staff to prepare for and possibly prevent their eventuality.

At the very least, a thorough preoperative assessment will alert the surgical staff to anticipate a complication, recognize early signs, and act in a timely and appropriate fashion to correct the problem, allowing the surgeon the opportunity to salvage a potentially life-threatening situation.

PATIENT EVALUATION
History
A thorough history needs to be obtained on each surgical patient. This history needs to include such things as presence of underlying illness, previous

E-mail address: dlw522@aol.com

0029-6465/06/$ – see front matter
doi:10.1016/j.cnur.2006.01.005

anesthetic experience, drug use, and allergies. A review of cardiac and pulmonary systems is critical to the successful administration of anesthesia and completion of the surgical procedure (Box 1).

Box 1: Emergency therapy for malignant hyperthermia

Cardiac system

Exercise tolerance

Angina, myocardial infarction

Symptoms of congestive heart failure

Arrhythmias

Valvular disease

Hypertension

Transient ischemic attack, cerebral vascular accident

Pulmonary system

Exercise tolerance

Obstructive versus restrictive disease; results of pulmonary functions tests and arterial blood gases (if indicated)

Baseline pulmonary examination, wheezing or rhonchi

History of bronchospasm, use of bronchodilators and/or corticosteroids

Recent pulmonary infections

History

Previous anesthetics

Previous complications

Allergies and adverse effects

Medical status

Family history

History of anesthetic related problems (malignant hyperthermia, nausea)

Medical diseases

Medications

Most drugs should be continued up to the time of surgery.

Some medications can have an effect on anesthesia management, such as central nervous system depressants, psychotropic drugs, diuretics, corticosteroids, and insulin

Smoking history

Presence of bronchospasm, chronic obstructive pulmonary disease

Change in sputum characteristics [2]

Physical Examination

A comprehensive physical examination should be completed. Attention to certain details is important (Box 2).

DEEP VEIN THROMBOSIS/VENOUS THROMBOEMBOLISM

Venous thromboembolism is a concern in the intraoperative and immediate postoperative phases of the surgical intervention. Certain types of surgery carry a greater risk for thromboembolism and thus make the need for thromboembolism prophylaxis necessary.

The risk of deep vein thrombosis (DVT) in general surgery patients is 25% to 30% without prophylaxis. That risk goes up to 70% following some orthopedic procedures without prophylaxis. Patients at risk for DVT are classified into three groups: low-risk, moderate-risk, and high-risk (Box 3) [3].

There are two foci addressed when looking at DVT prophylaxis: venous stasis and coagulation defects. Venous stasis is treated with graduated

---

Box 2: Risk factors for developing respiratory complications

Airway
Assessment of patient's neck, noting length, flexion, extension.
Assessment of patient's mouth, dentition

Cardiac system
Congestive heart failure
Arrhythmias
Diminished cardiac reserve/output

Pulmonary system
Wheezes
Rales
Rhonchi
Labored breathing (shortness of breath)

Body Habitus
Physical deformity/limitations
Obesity

Neurology (baseline neurological exam necessary on all patients who will undergo anesthesia [2])
Cranial nerves
Motor function
Muscular movements

Box 3: Breakdown of deep vein thrombosis risk in general surgery patients

Low-risk

Minor surgery (less than 30 minutes) with no factors except age

Major surgery (longer than 30 minutes), age older than 40 years, with no other factors

Minor trauma or medical illness

Moderate-risk

Major surgeries (urologic, gynecologic, general, vascular, neurologic, cardiovascular), age older than 40 years, or other factors

Major medical illness (cancer, heart/lung disease, inflammatory bowel disease)

Major trauma (third-degree burns)

History of DVT, pulmonary embolus, or thrombophilia

High-risk

Fractures or major orthopedic surgery (pelvis, hip, lower limb)

Metastatic disease

Major abdominal or pelvic surgery for cancer

Major trauma, illness, and surgery in patient with history positive for deep vein thrombosis, pulmonary embolus, or thrombophilia

Stroke or paraplegia with lower limb paralysis

Amputation or lower limb

compression stocking, elastic stockings, or simply encouraging the postoperative patient to ambulate early in the recovery process [3].

Elastic stockings provide consistent external compression along the entire length of the stocking and have been used to treat varicose veins for a long time. In the prophylactic treatment of DVT, elastic stockings have been replaced with intermittent pneumatic compression devices. Table 1 discusses the indications for DVT prophylaxis based on the risks to the patient [3]. Coagulation defects often are treated with anticoagulants such as traditional heparin therapy or low molecular weight heparin (LMWH).

Signs and Symptoms

Signs and symptoms of DVT include heat, redness, edema, pain in the calf, or a positive Homan's sign [4]. Diagnosis is usually accomplished with venous ultrasound.

Treatment

Anticoagulation is the mainstay of DVT treatment. The purpose of anticoagulation is to: prevent formation of new thrombus, prevent pulmonary embolism,

Table 1
Indications for deep vein thrombois prophylaxis

Risk	Indication
Low risk	Graduated compression stockings only
Moderate risk	Graduated progression stockings in conjunction with anticoagulants
High risk	Graduated progression stockings in conjunction with anticoagulants

Data from Evans D, Read K. Graduated compression stockings for the prevention of postoperative venous thromboembolism. Best Practices 2001;5(2):1–6.

and allow autogenous circulating thrombolysis to occur [5]. Box 4 discusses the duration of treatment for DVT [5].

The newest modality for treating DVT is LMWH. LMWH has many advantages compared with heparin:

1. Twice the half-life (4 hours)
2. 90% bioavailability when injected subcutaneously
3. Complication profile significantly less than heparin with relation to thrombocytopenia and bleeding
4. Single daily dose is possible
5. Complications of recurrent thromboembolism, death, and major bleeding less than with heparin
6. Decrease in mortality

Box 4: Duration of anticoagulants for deep venous thrombosis

Less than 6 months
First event
Reversible risk factors (surgery, trauma)

More than 6 months
First or several events with:
- Malignancy
- Anticardiolipin antibody
- Antithrombin deficiency
- Diagnosed thrombophilia

Lifetime
Multiple thrombophilic states
Multiple deep venous thrombosis events

Data from Sparks SR, Bergan J. Deep vein thrombosis. In: Cameron JL, editor. Current surgical therapy. 8th edition. Philadelphia: Elsevier; 2004. p. 869–71.

7. Cost effective because of lack of need for monitoring, no initial hospitalization needed, and fewer complications requiring recurrent hospitalization [5]

HYPOTHERMIA

Hypothermia is defined as a body temperature less than 36° C (96.8° F). As many as 60% of the patients admitted to the postanesthesia care unit (PACU) are believed to be hypothermic [6].

Preventive measures to decrease heat loss in the operating room (OR) include: maintaining an adequate temperature, providing warm blankets on arrival, and minimizing exposure by adequately covering the patient. Anesthesia also can use humidifiers, fluid warmers, and forced-air devices [1].

Patients with hypothermia have temperatures less than 36° C (96.8° Fahrenheit), which can induce shivering. Shivering increases oxygen demand by 300% to 400%. Therefore, oxygen therapy should be initiated and maintained in the postoperative period if necessary. Oxygen saturation also should be monitored [6].

EFFECTS OF HYPOTHERMIA
Hypovolemia
Vasoconstriction caused by hypothermia can cause intravascular volume loss and contribute to a fluid shift from the extracellular space. Upon rewarming, vasodilatation ensues, and the patient may require large amounts of fluid to avoid hypovolemia [6].

Central Nervous System Depression
The anesthetized patient with a temperature less than 96.8° degrees Fahrenheit will recover from anesthesia more slowly than a warm patient. Hypothermia delays metabolism and alters the effects of some types of anesthetic agents [6].

Clotting Abnormalities
Hypothermia decreases platelet activity and increases fibrinogen. These two factors combined increase the tendency for postoperative bleeding [6].

HYPERTHERMIA
The postoperative patient's temperature may be elevated as a result of an infectious process, sepsis, or a hypermetabolic process known as malignant hyperthermia (MH).

Malignant Hyperthermia
MH is a life-threatening emergency that is transmitted genetically as an autosomal-dominant trait. It is triggered by inhalation anesthetics and the depolarizing muscle relaxant, succinylcholine [6].

Incidence is 1:50,000 in adult anesthetics and 1:15,000 in children. The highest incidence is in patients who are younger than 15 years old, and incidence is greater in males than in females. Patients with central core disease and some muscular dystrophies are at an increased risk for MH (Box 5).

Once a patient has been identified as at risk for MH, the anesthesia provider must take appropriate measures. Box 6 outlines the Malignant Hyperthermia Association of the United States' emergency therapy for MH [6].

FEVER

Fever can be a response to infection or trauma, such as the trauma of surgery. Systemic inflammatory response syndrome (SIRS) is the febrile response that occurs after surgery. SIRS is defined by two or more of the following:

- Temperature above 100.2° Fahrenheit (38° C) or temperature below 96.8° F (36° C)
- Heart rate above 90 beats per minute
- Respiratory rate above 20 beats per minute or a Pa Co2 greater than 32 mm Hg
- White blood cell (WBC) count above 12,000/mm or below 4000/mm [7]

Sepsis is the systemic inflammatory response resulting from infection. The three most common types of postoperative infection are wound, urinary tract (UTI), and pneumonia.

Box 5: Signs and symptoms of malignant hyperthermia

Hypercarbia

Tachycardia

Tachypnea

Cardiac arrhythmias

Hypoxia and dark blood at the surgical field

Hypertension or unstable blood pressure

Muscle stiffness or rigidity

Mottling, cyanosis

Exhaustion of carbon dioxide absorbent

Hot absorption canister

Metabolic or respiratory acidosis

Rapid temperature increase (1° to 2° C every 5 minutes)

Myoglobinuria

Hyperkalemia, hypercalcemia, lactic academia

Pronounced elevation in creatinine kinase [6]

Prevention includes identifying patients with a predisposition for malignant hyperthermia.

Box 6: Emergency management of malignant hyperthermia

1. Immediately discontinue all triggering agents (inhalational anesthetics and succinylcholine).

2. Terminate surgery if possible, or continue with safe anesthetic drugs.

3. Hyperventilate with 100% oxygen at highest flow rate. It is not necessary to change any anesthesia equipment.

4. Immediately give dantrolene sodium 2 to 3 mg/kg intravenously. Give additional incremental doses up to 10 mg/kg total or until the signs of malignant hyperthermia are controlled.

5. Give sodium bicarbonate intravenously to correct the metabolic acidosis. Refer to arterial blood gas (ABG) values to determine dosage. If ABGs are not available, consider 1 to 2 mEq/kg.

6. If the patient is hyperthermic, begin active cooling.
   - Inject iced saline (not lactated Ringer's) intravenously 15 mL/kg every 15 minutes times three.
   - Used iced saline to lavage the stomach, bladder, rectum, and open body cavities as feasible.
   - Cool the body surface with a hypothermia blanket. Rub with cold, wet towels or ice.
   - Monitor the temperature to avoid hypothermia.

7. Cardiac dysrhythmias usually resolve with correction of acidosis and hyperkalemia. If not, antidysrhythmic agents such as procainamide 3 mg/kg (maximum of 15 mg/kg) may be used. Avoid calcium-entry blockers, because they may cause hyperkalemia and cardiovascular collapse.

8. Closely monitor temperature. ET CO_2 arterial or central venous blood gases, urine output K^+, Ca^{++}, and coagulation studies. Insert a urinary catheter. Consider arterial line and a central venous or PA catheter.

9. Hyperkalemia is common. Treat with hyperventilation, sodium bicarbonate, or 10 units of regular insulin in 50 mL of D_{50} intravenously titrated to K^+ level or regular insulin 0.15 units/kg in D_{50} 1 mL/kg. Life-threatening hyperkalemia also may be treated with calcium (eg, 2.5 mg/kg of $CaCl_2$).

10. Maintain urine output above 2 mg/kg/h. Consider volume of urine output to determine need for mannitol or furosemide.

11. Children younger than 10 to 12 years who have a sudden cardiac arrest without hypoxia after succinylcholine may have subclinical muscular dystrophy. Treat for acute hyperkalemia first. Give $CaCl_2$ with other treatments in step 9.

12. Transfer patient to the ICU when stable. Monitor at least 24 hours for recurrence of malignant hyperthermia (MH) and for late complications.

13. Administer dantrolene 1 mg/kg intravenously every 6 hours for 24 to 48 hours. Then dantrolene 1 mg/kg every 6 hours for 24 hours may be given orally as necessary.

14. Monitor core body temperature (continuously), ABG, K^+, Ca^{++}, creatine kinase (CK), serum and urine myoglobin, and coagulation studies until values return to normal.

15. Counsel the patient and family about MH and further precautions. Refer the patient to MHAUS and complete an Adverse Metabolic Reaction to Anesthesia report to the North American Malignant Hyperthermia Registry at 888-274-7899.

From DeLamar LM. Anesthesia. In: Rothrock JC, editor. Alexander's care of the patient in surgery. 12th edition. St. Louis (MO): Mosby; 2003. p. 248.

Wound Infections

The incidence of postoperative wound infections depends on type of surgery, length of surgery, use of prophylactic antibiotics, and whether the antibiotics are given at the correct time. Factors that increase the risk of infection in the surgical patient include: obesity, diabetes, use of steroids, length of hospitalization, preoperative underlying bronchitis, and prolonged postoperative ventilation.

Urinary Tract Infection

Urinary tract infection is more common in females than males. Patients who have Foley catheters placed, but especially patients who are catheterized for a prolonged period of time, are at an increased risk for UTI.

Pneumonia

Risk factors for postoperative pneumonia include age, chronic lung disease, and chest surgery. Mechanically ventilated patients are at an increased risk because of alterations in normal defense mechanisms such as cough. Patients may aspirate microorganisms from the oropharynx [7].

EVALUATION OF PATIENTS WITH POSTOPERATIVE FEVER

Assessment of signs and symptoms is focused on ascertaining system involvement. For example, the patient with a postoperative wound infection presents with erythema, pain at the surgical site, swelling, and decreased function caused by inflammation. The length, extent, and type of surgery affect the likelihood of an infection occurring [7].

Surgical procedures are classified as clean, clean contaminated, contaminated, and dirty. Surgical procedures classified as clean such as a breast biopsy are less likely to become infected than a contaminated case such as a ruptured diverticulum. Table 2 outlines the wound classifications [8].

The second most common postoperative infection, UTI, usually originates with an indwelling Foley catheter or from surgery on the urinary tract. Often these patients will have no signs or symptoms, but they may have lower back pain, lower abdominal pain, or flank pain. Diagnosis is obtained by urinalysis and urine culture [7].

The third most common postoperative infection is pneumonia. Patients at risk include those with prolonged intubation and those who have had surgery or anesthesia affecting the cough reflex or the cilia lining the respiratory cells [7].

Table 2
Wound classifications

Ia	Clean (hernia, varicose veins, breast)	Hollow viscus not entered (GIT, RT, UGT); no inflammatory processes
Ib	Clean prosthetic surgery (vascular grafts, orthopedic joint replacements, implants)	No break in aseptic technique
II	Clean–contaminated (cystoscopy, gastrectomy, elective open cholecystectomy)	GIT, RT, UGT opened without significant spillage
III	Contaminated (appendectomy, elective colorectal surgery, open/fresh accidental wounds, ruptured diverticulum of bowel)	Acute inflammation without pus; gross spillage from open viscus; major break in aseptic technique
IV	Dirty (fecal material abscess, peritonitis, old traumatic wounds, I & D, debridements)	Pus; perforated viscera; devitalized tissue present

Abbreviations: GIT, gastrointestinal tract; I & D, incision and drainage; RT, respiratory tract; UGT, urogenital tract.
  Data from Gruendemann B, Mangum SS. Infection prevention in surgical settings. Philadelphia: WB Saunders; 2001.

RESPIRATORY COMPLICATIONS

The potential for developing a respiratory complication postoperatively depends on numerous factors. These are listed in Table 3 [4].

According to Trayner, "the goal of preoperative assessment is to identify and modify risk factors for postoperative complications." Numerous interventions can be implemented preoperatively to impact the postoperative pulmonary function of the patient. These interventions include but are not limited to: smoking cessation, weight reduction, DVT prophylaxis, and coughing and deep breathing techniques [9]. Table 4 outlines the risks of postoperative respiratory insufficiency [10].

Table 3
Factors influencing postoperative complications

Preoperative	Pre-existing lung condition (asthma, emphysema, infection); smoking; chest wall deformity; obesity; extremes of age
Intraoperative	Types of preoperative medications; types and duration of anesthesia; types and duration of assisted ventilation; extent of surgical procedure
Postoperative	Shallow breathing; inability to cough; immobility

Data from Phillips N. Potential preoperative complications. In: Fortunato NH, editor. Berry and Kohn's operating room technique. 10th edition. St. Louis (MO): Mosby; 2004. p. 588–619.

Table 4 Risk of postoperative respiratory insufficiency	
Risk factors	Greatest risk
Age	Prematurity/infancy
	Elderly >70 years
Surgical type	Thoracic/upper abdominal
Duration of procedure	Greater than 2 hours[a]
Anesthesia setting	Emergency >8 pack years
Smoking history	
Active infection	Bronchitis or pneumonia
Cardiac disease	Congestive failure/shock
Chronic pulmonary disease	Hypercapnea/increased PVR
Neuromuscular disease	Weakness→hypercapnea
Malnutrition	Anergy/weakness
Obesity	>130 kg or ideal body weight + 100 lb
Hepatic disease	Active hepatitis or cirrhosis and ascit
Renal disease	Dialysis-dependant

[a]Duration of surgery has not been implicated in all studies.
From Watson CB. Respiratory complications associated with anesthesia. Anesthesiol Clin North America 2001;20(3):284.

ASPIRATION

Aspiration may occur intraoperatively because of decreased or absent throat reflexes. Gastric juices are highly acidic and very irritating to the lung parenchyma, potentially causing a chemical pneumonitis. Hypoxia results from edema formation, alveoli collapse, and ventilation–perfusion mismatch. Most aspirate is irritative, but it can be infectious if nasopharyngeal or gastric florae are involved [4].

There are certain patients who are poor risks for anesthesia. Two examples are patients who have not been NPO for at least 8 to 10 hours before surgery and patients with increased intragastric pressure. Increased intragastric pressure is seen in patients with intestinal obstruction, gastrointestinal bleeding and diaphragmatic hernia, and in other conditions. Inserting a naso–gastric tube before inducing anesthesia can reduce the risks of aspiration caused by increased intragastric pressure [4].

Signs and symptoms of aspiration include central cyanosis, dyspnea, gasping, and tachycardia. Without awareness and treatment on the part of the team, these could be followed by cardiac embarrassment, lung collapse, and lung consolidation.

Treatment

Treatment should be instituted within 5 minutes of aspiration to be the most effective. Most important is removal of as much aspirate as possible and limiting the spread of what is left in the lung. Maintenance of oxygenation is important, as is removal of carbon dioxide. There should be continuous monitoring of cardiac and respiratory status. Prophylactic antibiotics should be given if there is any risk of bowel contamination of the aspirate. A bronchodilator can be given to treat spasm [4].

LARYNGOSPASM AND BRONCHOSPASM

Laryngospasm is an involuntary partial or complete closure of the vocal cords. Bronchospasm is smooth muscle contraction that causes narrowing of the lumen in the bronchi and bronchioles. Oxygenation is difficult, as is carbon dioxide release, because airflow is decreased or possibly absent [4].

Signs and symptoms of laryngospasm include: wheezing, stridor, reduced compliance, central cyanosis, and respiratory obstruction [4].

Treatment

Treatment includes positive pressure ventilation, oxygenation, tracheal–bronchial intubation, and neuromuscular blockers for relaxation. Bronchodilators have direct effects on the heart, potentially leading to dysrhythmias or cardiac arrest. For this reason, they are given with caution. Patients also may be unresponsive to bronchodilators because of a disruption in their acid–base balance [4].

HYPOXIA/HYPOXEMIA

Hypoxia is a decrease in oxygen level in the arterial blood and tissues. Hypoxemia is decreased oxygen level in the arterial blood. Numerous factors are relevant to ensure adequate oxygenation. They are condition of the lungs, hemoglobin concentration, cardiac output, and oxygen saturation [4].

Hypoventilation has numerous causes, including pain, faulty positioning, alveolar impairment, a thick, short neck, or a full bladder. Central nervous system depression also will result in inadequate pulmonary ventilation [4].

The body compensates for a mild hypoxia by increasing heart and respiratory rates. The problem arises when the hypoxia progresses, and attempts at compensation become inadequate. Cardiac arrhythmia occurs, and irreversible damage to major organs of the body can be the ultimate result [4].

Signs and symptoms of hypoxia/hypoxemia include: increased pulse rate, increased respirations with decreased volume of the respirations, labored respirations, pallor or central cyanosis, and dark blood in the surgical field [4].

Treatment

Immediate oxygen administration is the treatment of choice for hypoxia, as well as postoperative coughing and deep breathing.

PULMONARY EMBOLI

Pulmonary emboli are usually blood clots that embolize in the pulmonary artery or one of its branches. Pulmonary embolism is a life-threatening process that is a major cause of death intraoperatively and in the immediate postoperative period [4].

The major cause of pulmonary emboli is venous stasis. Venous stasis is associated with obesity, congestive heart failure, and atrial fibrillation. If the patient is positioned on the OR bed for a prolonged period of time, blood flow to the lower extremities may be decreased by more than 50%, resulting in intra-operative venous stasis. This increases the need for instituting DVT prophy-laxis intraoperatively and postoperatively [4].

For patients at high risk for DVT, anticoagulation should be instituted as a preventive measure. The use of other modalities such as antiembolism stock-ings or an intermittent pneumatic compression device is also useful [4]. Signs and symptoms of a pulmonary embolus include:

- Dyspnea
- Pleural pain
- Hemoptysis
- Tachypnea
- Tachycardia
- Mild fever
- Persistent cough

A massive pulmonary embolus may be exhibited by:

- Air hunger
- Hypotension
- Shock
- Central cyanosis [4]

Treatment

Stabilizing the patient and gaining control of the situation is the first necessity. Treatments depend on the severity of the condition for each particular patient and include:

Bed rest
Oxygen therapy
Anticoagulation
Thrombolytic agents
Surgical de-embolization or placement of a vena cava filter [4]
Cardiac complications
Hypertension

HYPERTENSION

Patients who are at increased risk for intraoperative or postoperative hyperten-sion are those who were previously hypertensive and those undergoing specific vascular, thoracic, or abdominal surgeries. Surgeries that carry increased risk for developing hypertension include: carotid artery surgery, abdominal aortic aneurysm, peripheral vascular surgery, intraperitoneal surgery, and intratho-racic surgery [11].

Hypertensive events occur at four specific times intraoperatively:

- During laryngoscopy and induction of anesthesia
- Secondary to acute pain-induced sympathetic stimuli leading to vasoconstriction
- During postanesthesia phase 1 recovery
- 24 to 48 hours after surgery as fluid is mobilized from extravascular spaces [11]

Treatment

Treatment is aimed at prevention. Hypertension usually occurs as a result of withdrawal of a long-term antihypertensive regimen. The patient should be instructed to continue hypertensive therapy right up to the time of surgery. It should be reinstituted as soon as possible in the postoperative period. In the case of a hypertensive emergency (see Table 5), or if the patient cannot resume normal oral intake (see Table 6), parenteral antihypertensive therapy is indicated [11].

HYPOTENSION

Hypotension can cause myocardial ischemia, and it is a predictor of postoperative cardiac morbidity. The most common causes are intravascular volume depletion and excessive vasodilatation [11]. Hypotension occurs for numerous reasons in the intraoperative and postoperative phases of the surgical process. Anesthetic agents are major contributors to the onset of hypotension.

Diminished cardiac output and reduced peripheral resistance are effects associated with spinal or epidural anesthesia. An overdose of general or regional

Table 5
Drugs for treating perioperative hypertension

Drug	Administration	Dose range	Comments
Nitroprusside	IV	0.5–10 µg/kg/min	Requires invasive blood pressure monitoring; onset 2–4 min with brief duration of action; Use when urgent control of blood pressure required
Nitroglycerin	IV	20–400 µg/min	Useful with coexistent myocardial ischemia
Nicardipine	IV	Initiate at 5–15 mg/h; maintenance, 0.5–2.2 mg/h	Useful for patients receiving long-term calcium channel blockers
Fenoldopam	IV	0.1–0.3 mg/kg/min	
Enalaprilat	IV	0.625–1.25 mg every 6 hours	Useful for patients receiving long-term ACE inhibitors, angiotension receptor blockers
Labetalol	IV	20–80 mg as IV bolus every 10 min; up to 2 mg/min as IV infusion	Contraindicated in patient with excessive bradycardia or CHF
Esmolol	IV	25–100 µg/kg/min; may increase infusion rate to 300 µg/kg/min	
Methyldopa	IV	250–500 mg every 6 hours	Onset of action 4 h

Abbreviations: ACE, angiotensin-converting enzyme; CHF, congestive heart failure; IV, intravenous.
From Weitz HH. Postoperative cardiac complications. Med Clin North Am 2001;85(5):1154.

Table 6
Parenteral substitution of long-term oral antihypertensive therapy

Drug	Dosage
β-Blockers	
Propranolol	0.5–2.0 mg every 4–6 h IV
Labetalol	20–80 mg as IV bolus every 10 min; up to 2 mg/min as intravenously infusion
Esmolol	25–100 µg/kg/min IV; may increase infusion rate to 300 µg/kg/min
Diuretics	
Furosemide	20–60 mg IV
Central agent	
Methyldopa	250–500 mg every 6 h IV
Clonidine	Transdermal patch (must be placed 48 hours before desired effect)
Calcium channel antagonists	
Nicardipine	0.5–2.2 mg/h IV
Angiotensin-converting enzyme inhibitors, angiotensin receptor blocker	
Enalaprilat	0.625–1.25 mg every 6 h IV

Abbreviation: IV, intravenously.
From Weitz HH. Postoperative cardiac complications. Med Clin North Am 2001;85(5):1151–69.

anesthetic agents can occur. Unrecognized hypothermia with too much general anesthetic can lead to hypotension. Other causes of hypotension include:

- Volume depletion
- Circulatory abnormalities
- Cerebral or pulmonary embolism
- Myocardial infarction or ischemia
- Changes in patient position
- Excessive preanesthetic medication
- Epidural or spinal anesthesia above the level of T6
- Hypoxia
- Vagal response precipitated by intraperitoneal retraction [12]

Early signs of a hypotensive reaction or crisis include fluctuating and unstable blood pressure, vasoconstriction, and elevated serum pH or serum catecholamine. As the hypotensive state progresses, the following symptoms may appear: pallor or central cyanosis, clammy skin, dilated pupils, and decreased urinary output [12].

Treatment

The goal of treatment for hypotension is to restore adequate blood flow to the major organ systems. Measures such as placing the patient in Trendelenburg position and providing oxygen and rapid intravenous infusion to increase blood volume should be instituted. An early sign of hypotension is vasoconstriction (a physiologic response as the body attempts to raise the blood pressure). This can alert the anesthesia provider that blood pressure is low.

In certain situations, such as with spinal anesthesia, the patient's normal physiologic mechanism has been altered, and he or she is unable to vasoconstrict. Vasopressors that are designed to cause vasoconstriction of arterioles and veins while promoting myocardial contraction may be considered [12].

POSTOPERATIVE NAUSEA AND VOMITING

The incidence of postoperative nausea and vomiting (PONV) is 9% to 10% in the postanesthesia care unit (PACU). As the patient progresses through the first 24 hours, incidence increases to 30%. Surgical factors affecting PONV include surgical site and duration of the procedure. Certain patient specific-factors affect the incidence of postoperative nausea and vomiting. These include: age, gender, smoking, history positive for PONV, and motion sickness [12].

There are a few anesthesia-related agents that also have an effect on postoperative nausea and vomiting. They are opioids, nitrous oxide, propofol, and anticholinesterase drugs. Opioids are associated with a fourfold increase in PONV. Inadequate analgesia, however, is also a factor in PONV. Nonsteroidal anti-inflammatory drugs (NSAIDs), regional anesthesia, and liberal infiltration of local anesthetic all contribute to a decreased need for postoperative opioids, thus reducing the incidence of PONV [12].

The omission of nitrous oxide has been shown to decrease the incidence of PONV in procedures known to innately carry an increased risk. The decrease in symptoms may be related to a higher oxygen level and not necessarily to the use of nitrous oxide. Propofol, used for maintenance of anesthesia, has been shown to decrease PONV. It should be used with caution in the debilitated or elderly patient, however. Its effect is short-lived, with a half-life of 30 to 90 minutes. It has no analgesic properties, but when used in combination with another agent such as fentanyl, it lasts about 6 hours [12]. Anticholinesterase agents should be avoided, as they increase gastric motility and also may increase PONV. The effects of an anticholinesterase also may be dose-related [12].

Treatment

Goals of antiemetic therapy include reducing PONV, decreasing the length of hospitalization, reducing costs, and increasing patient satisfaction. PONV can be treated prophylactically or once symptoms have begun

Prophylactic PONV treatment has shown to enhance patient satisfaction; it includes avoiding general anesthesia if possible. If that is impossible, a multimodal approach to general anesthesia should be considered, with the use of propofol as a maintenance drug, and avoidance of muscle relaxants and nitrous oxide. A triple combination of droperidol (tranquilizer), dexamethasone (steroid), and ondansetron (antiemetic) should be administered at the end of the surgical procedure [12].

Treatment of PONV once it has occurred includes administration of ondansetron 1 mg intravenously. Ondansetron 1 mg has been shown to be as

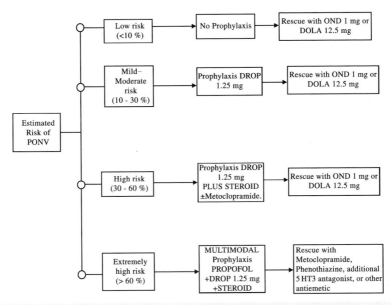

Fig. 1. Guidelines for the prophylaxis and therapy of postoperative nausea and vomiting (PONV). A low, mild, moderate, high and extremely high risk for PONV is determined by the presence of 0, 1, 2, 3, or 4 of the following factors, respectively: female gender, non-smoker, previous PONV/motion sickness, or opioid use. DOLA, dolasetron; DROP, droperidol; OND, ondansetron. (*From* Watcha MF. Postoperative nausea and emesis. Anesthesiol Clin North America 2002;20(3):709–22.)

effective as 2 to 4 mg in patients who have not received prophylactic treatment [12] (Fig. 1).

LATEX ALLERGIES

Latex allergy can be serious problem for operative patients and personnel when it occurs. It comprises about 10% of all life-threatening anaphylactic reactions that develop during anesthesia and surgery.

There two groups that are at an increased risk for latex allergy: health care workers and compromised patients. Table 7 outlines the groups most at risk for latex allergy and quantifies their risk [6,13]. Signs and symptoms include: urticaria, wheezing, dyspnea, laryngeal edema, bronchospasm, tachycardia, angioedema, hypotension, and cardiac arrest.

Treatment of Anaphylaxis

Management of latex allergy anaphylaxis includes stopping the anesthetic agent and giving pure oxygen, removing latex gloves and other items containing latex from the surgical field, and infusing intravenous fluids to sustain blood pressure. Epinephrine 3 to 4 *ug*/kg bolus augmented by an infusion of 1 *ug*/kg/min can be given if necessary [6].

Table 7	
Risk of latex allergy	
Group	Risk
Dental personnel	13.7%
Physicians (anesthesiologists, radiologists, surgeons)	9.9%
Perioperative personnel	2.5% to 15.8%
Perioperative RNs	10% to 7%
Hospital workers	1.3%
Other RNs	8.9%
Workers in the rubber industry	10%
General public	0.08% to 6.5%
Spina bifida patients	35% to 70%
Patients allergic to balloons, rubber gloves, certain foods or fruits	35% to 83%

Data from Rothrock JC, editor. Alexander's care of the patient in surgery. 12th edition. St. Louis (MO): Mosby; 2003.
Association of Operating Room Nurses.
AORN Standards, recommended practices, and guidelines. Denver (CO): Association of Operating Room Nurses; 2005.

Postoperatively, the patient should go to the ICU for observation for 24 to 48 hours. There should be careful observation of the airway, because there can be some laryngeal edema with the potential for recurrent laryngospasm and obstruction [6].

FOLEY CATHETERS

Troubleshooting a Foley catheter that is not draining postoperatively is a challenge for the postoperative nurse. It has been associated with numerous problems, including:

1. Low urine output as a result of dehydration, hemorrhage, or acute renal failure
2. Obstruction/blockage caused by kinking, stone debris, clots, or tissue fragments
3. Improper placement (This is problem is more common in males. Alterations to the urethra, either by trauma or otherwise, can result in the Foley being positioned in the urethra instead of the bladder. The catheter in some instances can even be passed into the periurethral tissue outside of the normal urethra.)
4. Bladder spasm (This can be exhibited by severe suprapubic pain. Bladder spasms can cause leakage around the Foley catheter. Spasm may be the only complaint, or it may be so severe that it obstructs urinary flow.)
5. Bladder disruption (If the bladder is severely distended secondary to a blocked catheter, this can result).
6. Balloon does not deflate [14]

Physical Examination of the Patient

Record the patient's vital signs to rule out hypovolemia looking specifically for tachycardia and hypotension. Assess the abdomen for bladder distention. Assess the patient's genitalia for bleeding, which can indicate trauma to the urethra.

Treatment

To assure that the catheter is functioning, attempt to irrigate it. A catheter that will not irrigate is probably not in the bladder but in the urethra. Using aseptic technique, gently irrigate the bladder with a 60 mL Toomey syringe and sterile normal saline. If the catheter cannot be flushed, it should be replaced [14].

An anuria workup will be necessary if the catheter flushes freely. Bladder spasms are treatable with oxybutynin, propantheline, or belladonna and opium supprettes. If attempting to remove a Foley catheter and the balloon will not deflate, instillation of 5 to 10 cc of mineral oil into the injection port will cause rupture of the Foley balloon in 5 to 10 minutes. Follow-up cystoscopy may be necessary to ensure that there are no balloon pieces retained in the bladder [14].

PAIN

All types of surgical procedures generate some type of pain. In fact, it is one of the major morbidities in the surgical patient. Adequate attention to management of postoperative pain may minimize or even eliminate numerous postoperative complications. By allowing the patient to ambulate earlier, minimizing catecholamine release, and avoiding postoperative hypoventilation, the patient's postoperative course can be eased significantly [1]. Nurses can control pain more effectively once they become attuned to picking up on cues the patient may send unconsciously [15].

There are numerous reasons for the presence and degree of surgical pain. For example, the patient who has abdominal surgery may have muscle pain secondary to the use of certain types of retractors. The patient who has had a gynecologic procedure in the lithotomy position may have hip, groin, or leg pain. The article on patient positioning (also in this issue) will discuss different surgical positions and the resulting issues associated with them more thoroughly. There are many modalities available to treat postoperative pain that include but are not limited to medication, regional blockade, and epidural analgesia.

Medication

Morphine is the most common medication used for major surgery. When used appropriately in small doses, it is a safe and effective drug. There are, however, adverse effects such as sedation, respiratory depression, nausea and vomiting, depression of cough reflex, and decreased gastric motility. These complications decrease the efficacy of morphine and allow an opening for less toxic medications to be used [1]. One of those less toxic medications, acetaminophen, is a simple analgesic that is essentially adverse effect-free. When used in combination with other drugs such as codeine or NSAIDs, it can be quite an effective analgesic. NSAIDs, another class of less toxic medications, can be used alone or in combination with a simple analgesic. They have been shown to have an opioid-sparing effect after major surgery [1].

Regional blockade

As an adjunct to general anesthesia, regional blockade provides pain relief in the immediate postoperative period and even longer if an indwelling catheter (as a regional anesthesia delivery system) is placed. Maximum doses of local anesthetics are listed in Table 8.

Epidural Analgesia

Epidural analgesia has become the gold standard for postoperative pain relief in patients who have had major surgery. It allows a pain-free immediate postoperative period, encouraging early mobilization. Additionally, patients have fewer postoperative pulmonary complications, and they improve gut function more rapidly following intra-abdominal surgery [1].

Nonpharmacologic Management

Methods of distraction and relaxation serve well as techniques to augment the use of analgesia, and they may decrease the amount needed by the patient. Studies have shown benefits to the patient following hysterectomy, major abdominal surgery, chest tube removal, and coronary artery bypass. Teaching these strategies preoperatively further increases the chance for an improved outcome. Hypnosis also has shown beneficial effects through decreased anxiety, decreased pain, reduction in analgesic need, and overall patient satisfaction. Acupuncture is becoming more accepted as a valid method for reducing the incidence of nausea and vomiting, and for pain reduction. Decreasing the requirement for pharmacologic intervention also results in a decrease in the possibility of adverse effects [16].

Applications of cold can reduce the pain threshold, decrease local inflammation and swelling, decrease tissue metabolism, alter the bleeding mechanism, and prevent or control muscle spasm. Cold has been especially effective following orthopedic and dental procedures. If implemented, cold should be applied immediately postoperatively in the recovery room and continued for 24 to 72 hours, depending on the extent of surgery and area involved.

Heat also may be used in conjunction with other therapies, and it usually is initiated 48 hours following surgery. In some situations, however, it may prove more effective if applied as soon as possible, as in renal colic following stone extraction or stent insertion.

Massage therapy, myofascial release, and positioning techniques all serve as viable adjuncts to standard pain management. Early ambulation and exercise not only reduce the risk of thromboembolism, but are effective for decreasing joint and back pain. Physical therapy may be added later in the patient's recovery.

Table 8	
Maximum doses of local anesthetics	
Drug	Dosage
Lidocaine (plain)	3 mg/kg
Lidocaine (with epinephrine)	7 mg/kg
Bupivicaine (plain or with epinephrine)	3 mg/kg
Prilocaine	600 mg [1]

SUMMARY

Complications occurring in the intraoperative phase or the postoperative phase of the surgical process can be devastating to the surgical patient. It impacts the surgeon personally, the institution monetarily, and the patient through slower return to normal life and function.

The attentive nurse cannot necessarily prevent postoperative complications but impacts the patient significantly by constant assessment and early attention to physical details that could alert the surgical team to what ultimately could become a major surgical complication. Early diagnosis and management may make the treatment of certain surgical complications a seamless process.

References
[1] Leaper DJ, Peel ALG. Handbook of postoperative complications. Oxford (UK): Oxford University Press; 2003.
[2] Klingensmith ME, et al. The Washington manual of surgery. 4th edition. Philadelphia: Lippincott-Williams-Wilkins; 2005.
[3] Evans D, Read K. Graduated compression stockings for the prevention of postoperative venous thromboembolism. Best Practices 2001;5(2):1–6.
[4] Phillips N. Potential preoperative complications. In Berry and Kohn's operating room technique. 10th edition. St. Louis (MO): Mosby; 2004. p. 588–619.
[5] Sparks SR, Bergan J. Deep vein thrombosis. In: Cameron JL, editor. Current surgical therapy. 8th edition. Philadelphia: Elsevier; 2004. p. 869–71.
[6] Rothrock JC, editor. Alexander's care of the patient in surgery. 12th edition. St. Louis (MO): Mosby; 2003.
[7] Perlino CA. Postoperative fever. Med Clin North Am 2001;85(5):1141–9.
[8] Gruendemann B, Mangum SS. Infection prevention in surgical settings. Philadelphia: WB Saunders; 2001.
[9] Trayner E, Celli BR. Postoperative pulmonary complications. Med Clin North Am 2001;85(5): 1129–39.
[10] Watson CB. Respiratory complications associated with anesthesia. Anesthesiology Clin North America 2001;20(3):275–99.
[11] Weitz HH. Postoperative cardiac complications. Med Clin North Am 2001;85(5): 1141–54.
[12] Watcha MF. Postoperative nausea and vomiting. Anesthesiol Clin North America 2002;20(3): 471–84.
[13] Association of Operating Room Nurses. AORN standards, recommended practices, and guidelines. Denver (CO): Association of Operating Room Nurses; 2005.
[14] Lefor AT, Gomella LG. Surgery on call. 4th edition. Philadelphia: McGraw-Hill; 2005.
[15] Manias E, Bucknall T, Botti M. Nurse's strategies for managing pain in the postoperative setting. Pain Manage Nurs 2005;6(1):18–29.
[16] Barson PK, et al. Options for postoperative pain management. Available at: www.guidelines.gov/summary/summary.aspx?doc_id=3284&nbr=2510.

Nurs Clin N Am 41 (2006) 173–192

NURSING CLINICS
OF NORTH AMERICA

Positioning Impact on the Surgical Patient

Mary Patricia O'Connell, CRNA

Department of Anesthesia, Paoli Hospital, 255 West Lancaster Avenue, Paoli, PA 19301-1792, USA

With the increased use of sedation in areas outside of the operating room, a greater understanding of the considerations and consequences of patient positioning is of growing importance. The experience of positioning patients in the operating room provides an excellent blueprint for these situations as well as increase the understanding how positioning can impact the postoperative care of surgical patients.

Articles on the subject of patient positioning during surgery use a wide variety of terms to describe these positions. Medical texts have adhered to the tradition of using Latin-based terms to describe patient's positions [1]. The word *decubitus*, from the Latin *decumbere* meaning "to lie down," is used as the base word, with additional descriptors added to indicate the part of the body in contact with the bed [2]. *Dorsal decubitus* means the patient's dorsal surface (their back) is in contact with the bed surface [3]. Simply stated, the patient is supine. Some medical texts, such as *Miller's Anesthesia* [4], are using more common terms such as *supine* and *prone*.

In describing a patient's lateral position for a left-sided procedure, the patient's right side is in contact with the bed and therefore could be described as *right lateral decubitus* or *right lateral* [1,3,4]. With justified emphasis on the correct procedure, the correct side, and the correct patient, some anesthesia practitioners have begun to record lateral and which side is up. Using this method, a patient scheduled for a right-sided procedure would be recorded in the lateral position with the right side up. Regardless of the terms used, the anesthesia record should provide a clear and accurate description of the patient's position during the surgical procedure and any changes made throughout the surgical course.

Although the surgical procedure dictates the patient's position, the surgeon's preference also plays a major role in positioning. For instance, hip procedures can be performed in either the lateral or supine position. The surgeon's physical comfort and skill at performing the procedure in a specific position are the

E-mail address: mpocs@mac.com

0029-6465/06/$ – see front matter
doi:10.1016/j.cnur.2006.01.010 nursing.theclinics.com

determining factors. Positioning is also often a balance between the position a patient can physically assume and physiologically tolerate [5]. Factors that limit patient positioning include

- Preexisting conditions (eg, arthritis)
- Decreased range of motion
- Previous surgical procedures
- Presence of a joint prosthesis
- Fractures
- Patient's age, height and weight [6]

These factors are assessed in the preoperative interview process [7]. The evaluation must be completed before the patient has been sedated. The nurse should also determine if the patient's hands and arms occasionally "fall asleep," if they have a "stiff" neck, or if they have back or leg. The nurse must explain to the patient how the positioning and anticipated duration of the surgery can impact these preexisting conditions and what measures will be taken to minimize exacerbation of these conditions.

Anesthesia impacts the positioning in several important ways. The nurse must first understand that regardless of whether a general, regional, or intravenous sedating technique is used, anesthesia blocks a patient's response to pain and pressure. These receptors are one of the body's greatest protective mechanisms, preventing overstretching and twisting of ligaments, tendons, and muscles [8]. By blocking these receptors that are sensitive to pain and pressure, patients undergoing anesthesia are vulnerable. Through careful preoperative examination and questioning; knowledge of the surgeon's positioning requirements; and knowledge of the impact of the anesthetic techniques, nurses can plan and carefully implement a comprehensive care plan for patients. Secondly, some of the effects anesthetics have on patients must be understood before specific positions can be discussed.

All anesthetic agents act to depress the autonomic nervous system, resulting in some degree of vasodilatation that is reflected in a lowered blood pressure. Changing the position of a patient undergoing anesthesia, regardless of what anesthetic technique is used, can make this decrease in blood pressure more profound. This drop in blood pressure is also affected by the preanesthetic volume state. The chronic use of diuretics and antihypertensives; bowel preparatory regimes; poor nutritional state; nausea and vomiting; and the presenting surgical condition can leave the patient in a volume-contracted condition [1,5]. Decreased tissue perfusion is always the result of a drop in blood pressure. The effect of vasopressors and especially the cold operating room environment compound the decreased perfusion [6].

These physiologic effects of anesthesia leave a patient more vulnerable to the effect of pressure. The effect of pressure on skin is important to understand. Pressure is exerted on the skin, soft tissue, muscle, and bone through the individual's weight against the surface of the bed (Fig. 1) [2]. As capillary perfusion pressure is approximately 32 mm Hg, any pressure above this

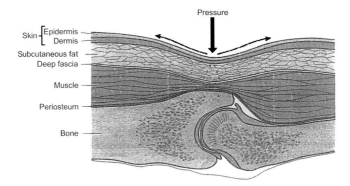

Fig. 1. Pressure on skin overlying a bony prominence is at greater risk for tissue damage. (*From* Phillips N. Berry & Kohn's operating room technique. 10th edition. St. Louis (MO): Mosby; 2004. p. 476; with permission.)

level exerted against the skin interferes with tissue perfusion. Most tissue can withstand pressures in excess of this for only brief periods. Prolonged exposure to pressures slightly in excess of this filling pressure initiates cascading events resulting in tissue ischemia, which leads to tissue anoxia and necrosis [2,5].

Certain conditions make the patient more vulnerable to the effect of pressure, including cardiac disorders, peripheral vascular disease, respiratory disorders, diabetes, advanced age, fractures, poor nutritional status, cancer, and neurologic disease [5,9].

The skin of older individuals is particularly vulnerable to injury. Their skin is less elastic and their dermis is thin and has less collagen, muscle, and adipose tissue compared with those of a young adult. These changes leave the skin more susceptible not only to pressure but also to bruising and skin tears, infection, impaired thermoregulation, and slow healing [9].

A staging system proposed by the National Pressure Ulcer Advisory Panel, which was subsequently outlined by Dharmarajan and Ahmed [10] and is presented in Box 1, provides guidelines for the evaluation of pressure.

Many different sources of pressure can affect the patient in the operating room, including the pressure their body exerts against the surface they are resting on, equipment resting on their body, the edges of a positioning frame or bed, positioning devices such as leg holders, or a member of the surgical team resting on or leaning against them. When the patient lays in the supine position, the skin over heels, elbows, and sacrum are most vulnerable to the compression that occurs between the bones in these areas and the surface of the bed [5].

The duration of the surgical procedure is significant in estimating the risk for tissue damage. Goodman [11] cites research showing that procedures lasting longer than 2 hours increase the risk for tissue damage by 35% to 50%, and procedures lasting longer than 4 hours triple this risk. Procedures lasting longer

Box 1: Pressure tissue injury staging system

Stage I
Nonblanchable erythema of intact skin
Discoloration of skin, warmth, edema, or induration may be indicators in dark skin

Stage II
Superficial ulcers involving loss of the epidermis, dermis, or both
Ulcers can present as an abrasion, blister, or shallow crater

Stage III
Full-thickness skin loss involving damage to subcutaneous tissue
Skin loss extends down to, but not through, underlying fascia

Stage IV
Full-thickness skin loss with extensive tissue destruction
Necrosis of underlying muscle, bone, tendon, or joint capsule [10]

than 4 hours put even the healthiest patients at risk for tissue damage from un-relenting pressure. Duration of surgical procedures cannot be predicted with any degree of certainty. Estimates for a procedure may be made using the surgeon's established track record and the patient's medical history, but many other factors influence the flow of a procedure. Therefore, the positioning requirements of every patient should be treated as though the procedure would last several hours. Medical professionals must remember that anyone who has remained immobile for a length of time may have some degree of muscle soreness and joint stiffness. In the patient who has undergone surgery, these complaints may not be verbalized because the pain at the surgical site dominates all other discomfort.

On nursing units, patients who are immobile are turned at intervals of at least every 2 hours. This movement is rarely possible during surgery [5]. Repositioning of a patient's head, arms, or heels may be feasible, but significant repositioning is rarely an option. In the operating room, good positioning techniques and padding products may have the ability to reduce, but not eliminate, the effects of pressure [11].

Lastly, the impact of hypothermia in further complicating not only the effects of pressure but also the overall postoperative outcome for all patients must be realized. A fall in core temperature is common in all patients undergoing surgical procedures, regardless of anesthetic technique [12]. In an attempt to conserve the core temperature, the peripheral vessels constrict. With this vasoconstriction comes a decrease in oxygen delivery to the tissues, which makes a patient more susceptible to tissue-damaging effects of pressure.

Impaired white blood cell function increases a patient's vulnerability to infection. Other consequences of hypothermia include bleeding, cardiac instability, and impaired platelet function [13]. The use of a forced air warming blanket is advisable on all patients. Intravenous fluids can be warmed easily by inserting a fluid-warming coil or placing most of the intravenous tubing under the forced air blanket. When a patient experiencing hypothermia emerges from general anesthesia and begins to shiver, their tissue oxygen requirements can increase 200% to 500% [9]. In these instances, oxygen administration is necessary to help meet the increased oxygen requirements.

SUPINE POSITION

Almost every patient is anesthetized in the supine position and is repositioned after induction if necessary. This position is most frequently used for

- General surgery
- Reconstructive and plastic procedures
- All procedures involving the anterior chest, epigastrium, and pelvis
- Orthopedic procedures of the hand and forearm, and knees and feet
- Neurosurgical procedures involving the anterior cervical and cranial structures [6]

When a patient assumes the supine position from standing, they experience a decrease in heart rate, vascular resistance, and a decrease in functional residual capacity and total lung capacity. The supine position causes increased pressure on the skin over the sacrum, elbows, and heels. The ligaments of the vertebral column relax with anesthetic agents and can result in a backache. Pressure alopecia has resulted from pressure on the occiput, especially in the presence of hypothermia in prolonged cases [1,3,6].

Remaining in the supine position for a long period is uncomfortable for anyone. Special precautions, such as placing a pillow under the patient's knees, help reduce the backache. Using padded cushions or added foam pads under the patient's sacrum, elbows, heels, and occiput will add to the patient's overall comfort.

In the supine position the arms should be placed on padded arm boards. The arms should be positioned palm up, supinated, and gently secured to the arm board. The possibility of injuries to the radial and ulnar nerves by compression against the edge of the arm board or by an assistant leaning against the arm board is well documented. Injury to the brachial plexus exists with abduction greater than 90° (Fig. 2). For procedures on the upper chest and neck, the arms must placed at the patient's side, and the elbows, areas of the ulnar nerve, and hands must be protected using foam pads. The arms are then placed at the patient's side with the palms facing inward. A draw sheet is brought up over the arms and smoothly tucked under the patient's body (Fig. 3) [3,5]. This method prevents the arms from falling down outside the mattress, risking serious nerve and tissue damage.

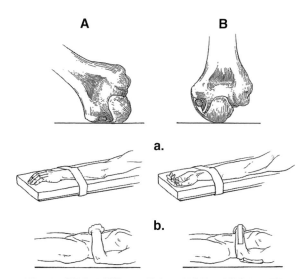

Fig. 2. The ulnar nerve at the cubital tunnel. *Column A* shows positions that threaten the nerve with compression. *Column B* indicates safer choices with supination or protective padding to lessen risks. (*From* Heizenroth PA. Positioning the patient for surgery. In: Rothrock JC, editor. Alexander's care of the patient in surgery. 12th edition. St. Louis (MO): Mosby; 2003. p. 167; with permission.)

The supine position can be modified to a contoured posture, which is referred to as *lawn* or *beach chair position,* and is frequently used for shoulder procedures [1,4]. This position can provide anterior and posterior access to the shoulder joint.

LITHOTOMY POSITION

The lithotomy position is required for combined abdominal and perineal; pelvic; and genitourinary procedures. Several types of lithotomy positions are possible, including standard (Fig. 4), low, and exaggerated (Fig. 5).

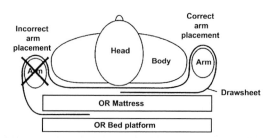

Fig. 3. Correct method for tucking arms at the patient's side. (*From* Heizenroth PA. Positioning the patient for surgery. In: Rothrock JC, editor. Alexander's care of the patient in surgery. 12th edition. St. Louis (MO): Mosby; 2003. p. 168; with permission.)

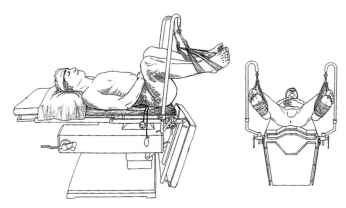

Fig. 4. Standard lithotomy position. Thighs are flexed slightly more than 90° on abdomen and knees are flexed enough to bring lower legs roughly parallel to the table. (Arms are not positioned correctly.) (*From* Warner MA, Martin JT. Patient positioning. In: Barash PG, Cullen, BF, Stoelting RK, editors. Clinical anesthesia. 4th edition. Philadelphia: Lippincott Williams & Wilkins; 2001. p. 643; with permission.)

All positions use some type of leg holder. Various leg holders are available and the selection should be based on the patient's anatomy and range of motion [1,3,5]. Standard and low lithotomy positions are used primarily when the surgeon requires access to the perineum and the abdomen, and for

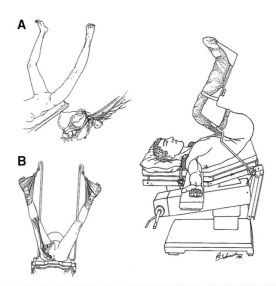

Fig. 5. The exaggerated lithotomy position. The pelvis is elevated and the legs aimed higher. (*From* Warner MA, Martin JT. Patient positioning. In: Barash PG, Cullen, BF, Stoelting RK, editors. Clinical anesthesia. 4th edition. Philadelphia: Lippincott Williams & Wilkins; 2001. p. 644; with permission.)

gynecologic procedures, sigmoid colectomy, and genitourinary procedures such as cystoscopy. The exaggerated lithotomy position is used for procedures that require transperineal access to the retropubic area, such as with a perineal prostatectomy [3].

The physiologic changes that occur with lithotomy will vary somewhat according to the leg position. These changes are primarily cardiac and respiratory. Raising the legs serves to "autotransfuse" the blood from the legs into the central circulation. This autotransfusion results in an increase in the cardiac output and venous return. The respiratory changes are caused by the increased intra-abdominal pressure limiting the movement of the diaphragm, resulting in decreased lung volumes. This increase in pressure is most marked in the exaggerated lithotomy and requires that ventilation be controlled [1,3].

The nerves that are most vulnerable in the lithotomy position are the common peroneal, obturator, saphenous, and femoral nerves. The legs should be positioned so that no part of the leg is resting against the leg holders. Care must be used in positioning the hips and knees to prevent an angle so acute that major vessels are compromised. The legs should be moved slowly and simultaneously into and out of the leg holders. This slow movement will allow the patient to physiologically adjust to the sudden shift in circulatory volume back into the legs. Administering additional intravenous fluids before returning the legs to supine position is frequently suggested to minimize the cardiovascular response [1,3,4].

The exaggerated lithotomy position is used for transperineal approach to the retropubic area. In addition to the standard lithotomy, the pelvis is elevated and the legs are flexed higher on the trunk. This elevation stresses the lumbar spine and stretches the lumbosacral muscles and ligaments. The perfusion of the legs and feet is dramatically reduced in this position and an increase in the pressure of the abdominal contents against the diaphragm occurs, mandating intubation and controlled ventilation [1,3,4].

Lengthy procedures in the exaggerated lithotomy have a high incidence of lower extremity compartment syndrome [1,3]. With the legs flexed on the trunk, the compression of muscles in the thigh can lead to edema. Because the fascial covering of muscles lacks elasticity, any edema puts more pressure on the muscle tissue, reducing perfusion and thereby increasing the ischemia and potentially leading to necrosis. These ischemic muscles release large amounts of myoglobin into the blood from the injured cells, resulting in renal damage and potential renal failure [1,4,14].

The arms may be positioned on padded arm boards, with the palms up and gently secured, or tucked. When the arms are tucked in any lithotomy position, some special considerations must be taken into account. With the arms tucked, the patient's fingers can migrate over the edge at the foot of the bed. The risk for trauma to the fingers is significant when the foot of the bed is raised [1,3,5]. The arms still must have the elbows protected with a foam pad and positioned with the palms facing in toward the body, but the hands must be enclosed and secured within a foam heel protector and the fingers prevented from slipping out.

LATERAL POSITION

The lateral position is used for orthopedic procedures involving the hip and, with some modification, for kidney and thoracic procedures. After regional or general anesthesia is established, the patient is carefully turned with the operative side up (Fig. 6). Enough people must be present to assist in turning the patient to prevent injury to the suprascapular nerve. A small roll is placed just below the axilla to lift the chest and relieve pressure on the axillary neurovascular bundle, allowing for adequate blood flow in the arm [1,3]. A pillow is placed under the patient's head to keep the cervical and thoracic vertebrae aligned while making sure that the dependent ear is not folded and is well padded. The eyes must also be protected and free from any pressure. The lower leg is flexed at the knee and a foam pad is placed under the head of the fibula to protect the peroneal nerve. The upside leg is extended and pillows are placed between the legs. The arms may be stabilized using one or two arm boards. If one lower armrest is used, pillows or folded blankets are placed between the arms to keep them in good alignment. If using two lower armrests, the lower arm is placed with the palm up. The upper arm should be on the same plane as the shoulder, with the forearm and wrist in a neutral functional position (Fig. 7).

The torso must be stabilized with all lateral positions. Padded braces or wide tape can be used to immobilize the patient. Tape is placed over the patient's shoulders and hip. Care must be taken that the shoulder tape does not prevent chest expansion and the hip tape does not lie over the head of the femur so snugly that the femoral head is compressed, which could result in aseptic necrosis [1].

When exposure is needed for renal or thoracic procedures, the lateral position is modified by flexing the bed so as to widen the intercostal spaces. For the

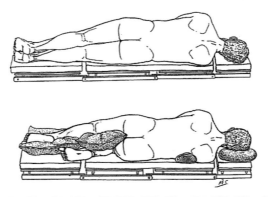

Fig. 6. The standard lateral position. Proper head support, axillary roll, and leg pillow have the vertebra in alignment. Not shown are the padding for the peroneal nerve and the securing straps. (*From* Warner MA, Martin JT. Patient positioning. In: Barash PG, Cullen, BF, Stoelting RK, editors. Clinical anesthesia. 4th edition. Philadelphia: Lippincott Williams & Wilkins; 2001. p. 650; with permission.)

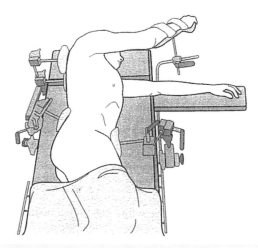

Fig. 7. Lateral with stabilizing braces and both arms supported on arm boards. (Lower arm should be supinated.) (*From* Phillips N. Berry & Kohn's operating room technique. 10th edition. St. Louis (MO): Mosby; 2004. p. 481; with permission.)

thoracic exposure, the lower part of the bed is flexed with the chest remaining level (Fig. 8). When access to the retroperitoneal area is required, the upper portion of the bed is also lowered and the "kidney rest" is raised (Fig. 9). The kidney rest is raised to increase the amount of flexion and improve exposure. The patient must be positioned so that the device is under the dependent

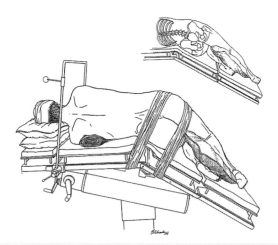

Fig. 8. The lateral jackknife position. Used to open intercostal spaces. Restraining tapes are properly placed. (*From* Warner MA, Martin JT. Patient positioning. In: Barash PG, Cullen, BF, Stoelting RK, editors. Clinical anesthesia. 4th edition. Philadelphia: Lippincott Williams & Wilkins; 2001. p. 653; with permission.)

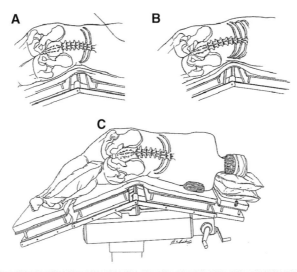

Fig. 9. The flexed lateral position for renal access. The two upper panels show improper placement of the kidney rest. The lower panel shows the rest at the correct point permitting the best expansion of the down side lung. (*From* Warner MA, Martin JT. Patient positioning. In: Barash PG, Cullen, BF, Stoelting RK, editors. Clinical anesthesia. 4th edition. Philadelphia: Lippincott Williams & Wilkins; 2001. p. 654; with permission.)

iliac crest. If the kidney rest is elevated and aligned under the patient's flank, ventilation of the dependent lung is severely restricted [1,3,5].

The pooling of blood in the lower extremities occurs in varying degrees with all lateral positions, and is greatest when the patient is flexed. The use of compression stockings will help minimize the systemic effect. In all lateral positions, the dependent lung receives a larger blood flow and the upper lung is easier to ventilate. This effect is referred to as a *ventilation-perfusion mismatch*. The presence of preexisting cardiac or pulmonary disease obviously decreases a patient's ability to tolerate all of these physiologic changes [1,3].

PRONE POSITION

The prone position is used for spinal procedures (including the cervical spine), accessing posterior cranial structures, certain orthopedic procedures (Achilles' tendon repair), and some rectal procedures. In this position, the patient's abdomen must be free from pressure because the increased pressure of abdominal contents restricts the movement of the diaphragm and, through a sequence of events, causes distended epidural veins. To minimize this occurrence, frames and various methods for supporting the patient's abdomen have been developed, each with its own merits.

Regardless of the type of support used, several factors in the planning and implementation of the procedure are consistent [1,3]. All equipment should be checked before anesthesia induction, ensuring that the frame or rolls are appropriate for the patient's size. Arm rests, head support, and all additional padding should be within easy reach [7]. Before a patient is positioned in the prone position, anesthesia should be induced and the patient intubated. After the airway is established and the endotracheal is secured, the patient's eyes must be protected. Protecting a patient's eyes is important with all general anesthetics and is usually accomplished by using tape or transparent adhesive dressing such as a Tegaderm (3M Health Care, St. Paul, Minnesota). Additional monitors; added intravenous lines; arterial lines; an esophageal stethoscope and temperature monitor; and urinary catheters are placed at this time. The turning and positioning sequence should be known by all participating in this process. Adequate manpower to turn and position is mandatory.

Many devices are available for positioning a patient in the prone position. Some devices are as simple as sheets or blankets tightly rolled to provide support from the patient's shoulder to just below their iliac crest, and others include several types of adjustable frames. Two distinct versions of frames are commonly used: the Wilson frame (Fig. 10), used for patients placed in a traditional prone position, and the Andrews frame (see Fig. 10), used for patients placed in a kneeling position. All frames should be well padded and capable of adjusting to fit the patient's body habitus. The surgeon chooses the type of frame used [5].

Regardless of the positioning device used, the abdomen must be free from any external pressure for all prone positions. If a patient lies on their abdomen,

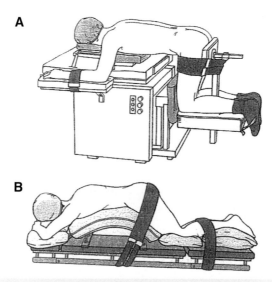

Fig. 10. Frames for spinal surgery. (A) Andrews frame. (B) Wilson frame. The arms in B are not properly positioned. (*From* Phillips N. Berry & Kohn's operating room technique. 10th edition. St. Louis: Mosby; 2004. p. 482; with permission.)

the intra-abdominal pressure is increased, resulting in venous engorgement. This engorgement ultimately results in venous congestion of the epidural veins [1,3]. Although this effect may be of only minor consequence with extremity procedures, it is of major importance for patients undergoing surgical procedures of the spine and cranium. Cutting these engorged vessels can result in rapid, massive blood loss. Keeping the abdomen free from pressure helps to minimize the risk for this type of blood loss [1,3].

Although the patient's head can be positioned and rotated to one side or the other, it is best to have the patient's head remain in the midline position. This position is particularly important when a patient has limited range of motion or a history of neck pain that may indicate a cervical disc [1,3]. Many commercial devices allow the patient's head to remain in the midline plane while keeping external pressure off of the eyes, providing a clear path for the endotracheal tube, and allowing a clear view of the patient's face and eyes. The P³ Prone Positioning Pillow (H.E.A.D. Prone, Inc., Cambridge, Massachusetts) has been used in the author's institution with a high degree of provider satisfaction (Fig. 11). If the patient is to be positioned with their head turned to one side, then a soft gel or sponge head support should be used, ensuring that the dependent eye is free from pressure and the dependent ear is well positioned and padded [1,3].

The arm position used in the prone position is chosen based on several factors, most importantly the surgeon's need. For procedures that require a fluoroscope, usually the patient's arms must be safely secured at their sides. When using a frame or rolls, the patient's arms must be elevated on blankets to remain in alignment with the body. The elbows and hands must be protected

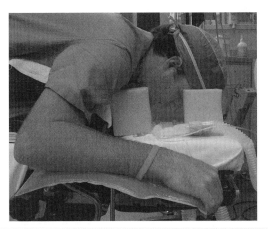

Fig. 11. P³ Positioning Pillow (H.E.A.D. Prone, Inc., Cambridge, Massachusetts) in use. Patient has eyes protected using Tegaderm (3M Health Care, St. Paul, Minnesota). The arms are in proper alignment. The Allen Prone Arm Support (Allen Medical Systems, Acton, Massachusetts) with its multiple adjustment joints allow for positioning to each patient's anatomy.

using foam pads and then placed with the palms facing in toward the thighs and secured. When securing the arms and hands, the hands and wrists must be kept aligned in a functional position [1,3]. If the arms are placed on arm boards, several options are available. A traditional well-padded armrest may be placed parallel to the operating room bed, or an armrest with multiple adjustment joints such as the one manufactured by Allen Medical Systems may be used. Regardless of the choice, several principles must be applied. The arms should be placed on the padded boards, ensuring that no muscles are under tension, the elbow is free from any pressure sources, and the forearm, wrist, and hand are neutral and in alignment. To avoid pressure of the humeral head on the axillary neurovascular complex, the arms must not be brought over the head. After the arms are positioned, pulses should be checked in both wrists [1,3].

Some believe the Andrews kneeling frame prevents pressure on the abdomen more successfully for patients who are obese than does the Wilson frames. However, patients who have existing knee conditions may develop problems in the postoperative phase when an Andrews frame is used, and this must be weighed against the potential benefits in the preanesthetic interview. The knees should be very well padded whenever this frame is used [1,3].

One of the most common physiologic changes accompanying the transfer from supine to prone position is hypotension. The hypotension that frequently occurs with induction of anesthesia is caused by loss of autonomic tone and may be magnified with the shift to the prone position. This effect can be more profound when using the Andrews frame because the legs are in a dependent position.

If the patient lies directly on their abdomen, the lung volumes decrease because of the hindered movements of the diaphragm. When the patient is in the supported prone position, where the abdomen is free from pressure, pulmonary compliance is near normal and the loss of functional residual capacity is less than in the supine or lateral position [1,3]. In fact, use of the prone position has been studied as a method for "recruiting" collapsed alveoli and improving gas exchange in acute respiratory distress syndrome (ARDS). Vollman [15] describes studies in which more than 70% of all evaluated patients who had ARDS responded to the prone position with an increase in PaO_2.

In the prone position, gravity causes an accumulation of extravascular fluid in any dependent extremity, including the hands, feet, face, and conjunctiva. The longer the procedure, the more dramatic the edema. This transient edema can exacerbate certain preexisting conditions, such as intermittent numbness in the hands. Patients should be advised to remove all rings and every effort must be made to remove all rings before surgery in these prone cases. For rings that cannot be removed without causing tissue damage, the patient must be notified that the ring may need to be cut off. This edema will also impact the nose and pharynx. Therefore, patients who have had lengthy procedures or those who have questionable airways may remain intubated for the immediate postoperative period [1,3].

Patients who undergo long procedures in the prone position are vulnerable to skin pressure injury. The knees, lower costal margins, and iliac crests are areas that are most susceptible to the effects of pressure in this position. In addition to the pressure in these areas, the small movements that occur with the insertion of spine-stabilizing hardware can also cause friction on the patient's skin [11]. In these types of procedures, applying a skin barrier film product such as Cavilon (3M Health Care, St. Paul, Minnesota), followed by Tegaderm or Tegasorb (3M Health Care, St. Paul, Minnesota), may be worth considering. In the author's institution, these products have been used on these areas for patients undergoing procedures lasting 8 hours, with no observed skin injury from pressure, friction, or shearing.

Patients have reported perioperative vision loss after undergoing spine surgery in the prone position [16], and after cardiac bypass and head and neck operations. The effect may range from loss of visual acuity to complete blindness. Reported causes include

- Central retinal artery occlusion
- Anterior ischemic optic neuropathy
- Posterior ischemic optic neuropathy
- Cortical blindness

Risk factors include

- Diabetes
- Hypotension
- Anemia
- Extended time in the prone position
- Large blood loss
- Fluid management
- Adverse drug effects
- Unique anatomic variations in the optic nerve blood supply [1,16]

Common variations of the prone position used in surgery include jackknife (Fig. 12) and prone with head up (Fig. 13). Jackknife is used to provide exposure to the sacral, rectal, and perineal areas. For general anesthetics, the patient's chest is elevated using chest rolls, or with pillows when a patient is having a regional anesthetic. A pillow is placed under the patient's hips, which are aligned with the break in the operating room bed. The bed is then flexed with the feet placed on a pillow to protect the toes. This position causes dramatic cardiac and respiratory physiologic changes, with the circulatory changes related to the dependency of the head and legs. When the abdomen and chest are elevated off of the bed surface, the head-down position pushes the abdominal viscera against the diaphragm, severely compromising respirations [1,5].

The prone head-up position is widely used to provide access to the posterior head and neck (see Fig. 13), and to replace the full sitting position (Fig. 14). In addition to the obvious cardiac and respiratory physiologic complications of postural hypotension that occur with the full sitting position, the risk for air

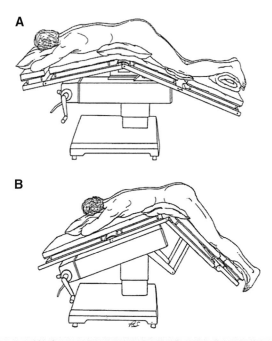

Fig. 12. The prone jackknife positions. (*A*) Low jackknife. (*B*) Full jackknife. (Arms are not positioned correctly.) (*From* Martin JT. Patient positioning. In: Barash PG, Cullen BF, Stoelting RK, editors. Clinical anesthesia. 2nd edition. Philadelphia: Lippincott Williams & Wilkins; 1992. p. 728; with permission.)

embolization presents potential lethal consequences. The opportunity for air to enter the circulatory system through an open vein in a surgical wound located above the heart increases in direct relationship to the elevation of the operative site. Although the prone head-up position significantly reduces this risk for air embolization, it does not eliminate the possibility [1,3].

When using the prone head-up position, the patient is intubated after anesthesia is induced, all monitors are applied, and a skull-pin–type head rest is placed on the patient (see Fig. 13). In an orderly and unified manner, the patient is turned and positioned on chest rolls to support the shoulders to just below the iliac crests while ensuring that the patient's abdomen is free from pressure [7]. The patient's elbows and hands are padded, placed at the patient's sides with the palms facing in toward the thigh, and secured. The height of the rolls may require folded blankets be used to keep the arms aligned with the patient's body. The patient's knees are resting on foam pads and lower legs are elevated on pillows.

FRACTURE BEDS

The fracture bed is a specialized positioning apparatus that requires a separate discussion. The fracture bed is used to position a patient for repair of a femoral

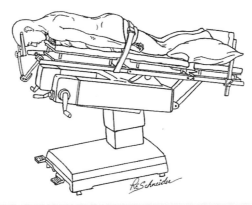

Fig. 13. The skull-pin head rest. Used to stabilize a patient in the head-elevated prone position. Patient is on chest rolls to free abdomen. Note the patient's arms are without protective padding and not in the proper position. (*From* Martin JT. Patient positioning. In: Barash PG, Cullen BF, Stoelting RK, editors. Clinical anesthesia. 2nd edition. Philadelphia: Lippincott Williams & Wilkins; 1992. p. 733; with permission.)

fracture and some types of hip fractures (Fig. 15). This bed permits the fractured leg to be placed to traction so that the bone fragments may be manipulated, realigned, and fixated using some type of hardware. The patient is anesthetized before being moved to this bed. The arm on the fracture side must be safely positioned over the patient's chest to permit the surgeon full

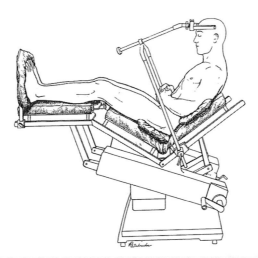

Fig. 14. Sitting position. This position provides access to the posterior cranial structures. With the surgical incision about the level of the heart the opportunities or air embolization are greatly increased. (*From* Martin JT. Patient positioning. In: Barash PG, Cullen BF, Stoelting RK, editors. Clinical anesthesia. 2nd edition. Philadelphia: Lippincott Williams & Wilkins; 1992. p. 732; with permission.)

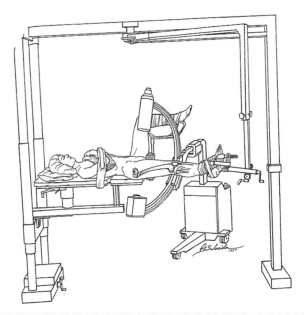

Fig. 15. The fracture bed. This device permits elongation of the fractured extremity allowing for the bone fragments to be repositioned. The opposite leg is elevated to provide for radiograph access to the fracture site. The arm on the side of the fracture is positioned over the patient's chest. (*From* Martin JT. Patient positioning. In: Barash PG, Cullen BF, Stoelting RK, editors. Clinical anesthesia. 2nd edition. Philadelphia: Lippincott Williams & Wilkins; 1992. p. 720; with permission.)

access to the fracture. A vertical pole is placed at the perineum. This pole must be well padded and is placed against the pelvis between the genitalia and the uninjured leg. If this is misplaced, damage can occur to the genitalia and the pudendal nerves. Other complications include brachial plexus injury and lower extremity compartment syndrome [4].

SUMMARY

The challenges of positioning and the accompanying physiologic risks are no longer isolated to the operating room. In areas such as interventional radiology, cardiac catheterization laboratories, and gastrointestinal suites, patients are being sedated with some of the same medications used for anesthesia, although perhaps in lower doses. The intention is for patients to remain immobile throughout the planned procedure. Although intensive care units have been using continuous intravenous sedation and muscle relaxants for some time, some of these units are now placing patients in the prone position to increase gas exchange for select patients who have ARDS [15]. Again, the intension is for patients to remain immobile throughout the planned procedure. Like surgical patients, these patients who are sedated and immobile are at increased risk for positioning complications. When a patient complains of pain in a location that does not seem to be related to the procedure, positioning during that procedure should be evaluated.

This article discusses many types of potential complications associated with patient positioning during surgery. It is important to understand that nerve damage is the second most common type of anesthetic complication represented in the American Society of Anesthesiologist Closed Claims Database. Ulnar neuropathies were the most frequent followed by brachial plexus. These complications are found in medical and surgical patients. The mechanisms for nerve injuries include stretch, compression, ischemia, metabolic derangement, and surgical injury. A certain threshold of pressure or duration of compression may be required to produce clinical symptoms. Conditions such as diabetes, malnutrition, cancer, smoking, alcoholism, previous nerve injuries, and extreme weight have been associated with an increased incidence of postoperative neuropathies [4]. Many of these patients are believed to have asymptomatic nerve conduction defects that become symptomatic during the perioperative period. Injuries discovered in the postanesthesia care unit are more likely to have occurred during the operative period, but those that have delayed onset (as long as 7 days) are more likely to have occurred during the convalescent period [1,3].

As this article has tried to emphasize, sedating patients places them at a greater risk for positioning complications. Nursing professionals have a presence within most of these patient care areas and must be the advocates for vigilance in this area of patient safety. The beauty of a perfectly performed procedure is dulled if the patient incurs an injury from poor positioning. All of the nursing staff's experience must be applied in properly protecting patients. When complications arise, constructive collaboration to find solutions and prevent recurrence is imperative. With the emphasis on safety and improving outcomes, all health care providers must be motivated to explore open communication between departments. Professional nurses who have different specialties have one important fact in common: they are the backbone of health care. They must ensure that this care is performed at the highest standard.

References

[1] Martin JT. Patient positioning. In: Barash PG, Cullen BF, Stoelting RK, editors. Clinical anesthesia. 2nd edition. Philadelphia: Lippincott Williams & Wilkins; 1992. p. 709–36.

[2] Revis DR, Caffee HH. Pressure ulcers, nonsurgical treatment and principles. Available at: http://www.emedicihe.com/plastic/topic424.html. Accessed August 20, 2005.

[3] Warner MA, Martin JT. Patient positioning. In: Barash PG, Cullen BF, Stoelting RK, editors. Clinical anesthesia. 4th edition. Philadelphia: Lippincott Williams & Wilkins; 2001. p. 639–65.

[4] Faust RJ, Cucchiara RF, Bechtle PS. Patient positioning. Miller's anesthesia. 6th edition. Philadelphia: Eisevier; 2005. p.1151–67.

[5] Heizenroth PA. Positioning the patient for surgery. In: Rothrock JC, editor. Alexander's care of the patient in surgery. 12th edition. St. Louis (MO): Mosby; 2003. p. 159–86.

[6] Phillips NF. Berry & Kohn's operating room technique. 10th edition. St. Louis (MO): Mosby; 2004. p. 470–91.

[7] AORN. Recommended practices for positioning the patient in the perioperative practice setting. Standards, recommended practices, and guidelines. Denver (CO): The Association; 2005.

[8] Guyton AC, Hall JE. Textbook of medical physiology. 10th edition. Philadelphia: Saunders; 2000.

[9] Dunn D. Preventing perioperative complications in an older adult. Holist Nurs Pract 2005;19:54–9.

[10] Dharmarajan TS, Ahmed S. The growing problem of pressure ulcers. Available at: http://www.postgradmed.com/issues/2003/05_03/dharmarajan3.html. Accessed August 21, 2005.

[11] Goodman T. Pressure damage in surgery. Available at: http://nursing.advanceweb.com/common/EditorialSearch/AViewer.aspx?AN=NW_05jul14_n2p33.html&AD=07-04-2005. Accessed September 26, 2005.

[12] Watters JM, McClaran JC, Man-Song-Hing M. The elderly surgical patient. ACS surgery: principles & practice. Available at: http://www.medscape.coom/viewarticle/508534. Accessed September 2, 2005.

[13] Welch TC. AANA journal course. Update for nurse anesthetists. A common sense approach to hypothermia. AANA 2002;70(3):227–31.

[14] Uratsuji Y, Ijichi K, Irie J, et al. Rhabdomyolysis after abdominal surgery in the hyperlordotic position enforced by pneumatic support. Anesthesiology 1999;91(1):310–2.

[15] Vollman K. Prone positioning in the patient who has acute respiratory distress syndrome: the art and science. Crit Care Nurs Clin North Am 2004;16(3):319–36.

[16] Lee LA. Perioperative visual loss: 31-year-old female scheduled for a redo spinal fusion with instrumentation. Available at: http://www.medscape.com/viewarticle/506675. Accessed August 17, 2005.

Nurs Clin N Am 41 (2006) 193–218

NURSING CLINICS
OF NORTH AMERICA

ELSEVIER
SAUNDERS

Comparison of Operating Room Lasers: Uses, Hazards, Guidelines

Phyllis M. Houck, RN, MS HEd, CNOR

Paoli Hospital, 255 West Lancaster Avenue, Paoli, PA 19301, USA

When Einstein formulated the theory of stimulated emission in 1917, it provided the foundation for laser technology. In 1958, Schawlow and Townes further investigated Einstein's theory and developed the principles of the laser. The first laser used in medicine and surgery was the ruby laser, and it was invented by Maiman in 1960. This laser was used for dermatological applications and for retinal photocoagulation in patients with diabetic retinopathy. Although this laser was not very efficient, it laid the groundwork for development of other lasers. Scientists soon discovered that other lasing mediums could be electrically stimulated to produce laser light in various wavelengths.

Another breakthrough in laser surgery occurred in 1972, when Jako adapted the CO_2 (carbon dioxide) laser for use on the operating microscope.

Other specialists soon followed, using the CO_2 laser in their own areas of expertise. In 1975, neurosurgeons were using the CO_2 laser to vaporize large tumors with minimum manipulation of the tumor, and in 1977, Bellina adapted the CO_2 laser for use in gynecology. The Nd:YAG (neodymium: yttrium-aluminum-garnet) laser in a pulsed modality also was introduced in 1977 and used in the fields of urology and gastroenterology by German physicians. In 1985, Jaffe and others revolutionized this laser when they adapted this modality to a contact laser using sapphire quartz probes [1].

With the growth of lasers around the world many countries established societies to promote and share information regarding lasers. In 1980, the American Society for Laser Medicine and Surgery was formed in the United States. Its goal is to unite health care providers in clinical laser applications, provide laser education, and promote laser research.

BASIC LASER BIOPHYSICS

The word LASER is an acronym and stands for light amplification by the stimulated emission of radiation. Information gathered from classical electromagnetic theory and atomic theory is needed as a background to understand lasers.

E-mail address: phyliscnor@aol.com

0029-6465/06/$ – see front matter
doi:10.1016/j.cnur.2006.01.004

Electromagnetic Waves

To a physicist, a wave is specified by four important characteristics: wavelength, frequency, velocity, and amplitude. The wavelength is the distance between any two successive crests, determining its color and measured in nanometers, while the frequency is the number of waves passing a given point per second. Velocity is the rate at which the wave profile moves forward, and amplitude is the magnitude of the vibrations, defined as the height of a wave crest. Light is a form of radiant energy or waves, that is, electromagnetic waves. The different forms of radiant energy can be classified by their wavelengths and arranged according in the electromagnetic spectrum. Table 1 shows the different kinds of electromagnetic energy according to their decreasing wavelengths. The energy of radiation is proportional to its frequency. People cannot sense the presence of radio waves even when close to an antenna of a powerful broadcasting station. The energy of ultraviolet waves, however, will become painfully evident to any one who sunbathes without sunscreen.

Atoms and Light Waves

To understand the laser, one needs to understand the atom and how it becomes laser light. All light is emitted by atoms, and there are rules that govern the way in which an atom absorbs and re-emits energy. Every atom has a certain energy state that it can occupy; when an atom absorbs energy, it moves to a higher energy state. Conversely, when it returns to a lower energy plane, it gives up energy or emits radiation. In simple terms, imagine an atom to be a coil spring; when there is no compression, it is in its ground or resting state. When the spring is compressed, however, it has added potential energy to the

Table 1
Surgical lasers on the electromagnetic spectrum

Ultraviolet	0.00001 nm	Cosmic rays	Short waves, high energy that can
	0.0001 nm	Gamma rays	break molecular bonds or damage
	0.1 nm	X-rays	molecules such as DNA or RNA
	10.0 nm	Ultraviolet	(ribonucleic acid)
	193 nm	Argon fluoride	
Visible	488 nm	Argon	
	514 nm		
	532 nm	KTP	
	632 nm	HeNe	
	694 nm	Q-switched ruby	Longer waves, lower energy,
Invisible	800 nm	Indigo	thermal effect of energy output
	850 nm		not enough to break molecular bonds
	1060 nm	Nd:YAG	
	2100 nm	Ho:YAG	
	2940 nm	ER:YAG	
	10,600 nm	CO_2	
	1.0 cm	Microwaves	
	100 cm	TV/FM radio	
	10,000 cm	AM radio	

system. When the spring is released, it bounces back and vibrates, giving up its kinetic energy [2].

The level in the system with the lowest energy is called the ground level, or resting state, every other level is an excited energy level. When an atom absorbs energy, it moves to a higher energy state, but when the atom returns to its ground level, it gives up its energy or photon. If this photon is close to another atom of equal energy and it is also in an excited state, it will interact with this atom, causing it to return to its resting state. Both atoms will give up their energy, and two identical photons will be emitted. This process is called stimulated emission of radiation. In lasers, the medium must have more atoms in the excited state versus the resting state, causing a condition called population inversion of the lasing medium; laser energy can now be discharged [3].

Laser Light

The laser light or beam has three unique characteristics that distinguish it from ordinary light. Laser light is monochromatic, meaning it is composed of photons of the same wavelength or color. Ordinary light contains many different wavelengths. Laser light also is collimated, consisting of waves parallel to each other. Light from other sources are noncollimated or spread out over a distance like light from a flashlight. Finally, laser light is coherent, meaning all the waves are orderly and in phase with each and do not diverge from one another as they travel in the same direction.

How Lasers Work

Laser light originates from a selected assembly of atoms, molecules, or ions, and it can be dispensed in several different media. Any selected substance capable of giving rise to a laser light is defined as a laser medium. Energy supplied to the medium is called pumping the medium, which now will be referred to as the active medium. The name of the laser usually is derived from the actual medium that caused the lasing action. The solid-state laser uses a solid matrix such as a crystal or glass. Gas lasers use a mixture of gases contained in a tube. Liquid lasers use complex organic dyes in a suspension or solution. The electronic laser, commonly referred to as diodes, use two layers of semiconductive material sandwiched together to produce low energy.

There are five essential elements to a laser system, the excitation source, laser head, ancillary components, control panel, and the delivery system. The excitation source provides the energy to the laser head, which in turn produces the laser light. This source can be electrical, chemical, flash lamps, or other laser systems. Next, the laser head houses the active medium, producing the photons or laser energy. Usually a system of mirrors, reflective and partially reflective, is the feedback mechanism needed to amplify the light produced by the stimulated emission of the laser light. The production of laser light also is aided by the ancillary components of the system such as the console. The console is the framework of the laser, and it protects the parts and laser components from damage. It also may house other items needed to run the laser, such as the cooling system or vacuum pump. All items housed in the console will be listed in the service manual of the laser. The fourth item of the laser system is the control panel, which allows the operator to select and use the full range of the laser's functions. This includes the power setting or wattage, time exposure, desired mode of application, and the emergency stop button. Computerization has allowed the control panel to be more user-friendly, and with the addition of the microprocessor systems to the laser, it allows the desired settings to appear with a mere touch of a button. The last part of the laser is its delivery system, which is the device or attachment that allows the laser energy to be transmitted from the laser head to the tissue. The laser energy can be delivered through a hollow tube with special mirror attachment called the articulating arm. This arm can be used freehand or attached to microscopes, slit lamps, colposcopes, and endoscopes. The second method of delivery is through a flexible fiber system.

Laser Power

Power density is the most important factor in the effective application of any laser. It determines the laser's ability to vaporize, excise, and coagulate. Power density is defined as the amount of power that is concentrated into a spot. Three variables determine the spot size of a laser beam. The first variable is the focal length of the lens, which affects the size of the beam spot. Second is the wavelength of the laser, which also limits the beam's focusing ability and size. Last is the transverse electromagnetic mode (TEM), which determines the precision of the spot by the power distribution over the spot area.

Fluence is a concept involving the power of the beam and is the amount of energy delivered to the tissue. It involves the power (watts), time, and spot size or area. If any of these parameters change, the tissue effects also will change. Excessive tissue damage can be avoided by using the highest appropriate wattage for the shortest period of time. Thermal tissue effect is determined by the amount of time that the laser beam is in contact with the tissue [3]. The control panel on the laser unit allows the user to enter the settings that will be the most efficient and appropriate for the procedure.

Laser–Tissue Interaction

When laser energy is delivered to tissue, an interaction occurs, and this depends on the type of tissue encountered and the wavelength of the specific laser being used. This knowledge will allow the perioperative nurse to prepare the appropriate laser for the procedure and be aware of any hazards that could present during the case. Reflective, scattering, transmission, and absorption are the four types of tissue interactions that can occur from the laser beam. When the laser beam leaves the surface and strikes at the same angle as it entered, it has been reflected. If the laser beam has been reflected in its entirety, it is called specular reflection, and this type of interaction is useful when dealing with tissue in hard-to-reach areas, such as vocal cords or ovaries. Diffuse reflection is the result of the laser beam being scattered. This occurs when the beam hits a curved surface of an instrument and is diffused and spread out over an area. Specialty coated or ebonized instrumentation can diffuse the laser beam further and decrease the amount of reflection that can occur at the surgical field. This would decrease the potential for damage that could be caused by the laser beam in the surgical field.

Scattering of the laser beam occurs when the distribution of the laser light energy within the tissue is altered, and the beam is scattered through the tissue. If this scattered energy is absorbed by the tissue, it is converted to heat. Care must be taken when using endoscopic instruments with certain lasers, because backscatter of the beam may occur, causing damage to the optics or distal end of the scope.

When the laser beam passes through tissue or fluids without thermally affecting the area, transmission of the laser beam has occurred. This interaction of the laser beam on tissue is important when the beam must pass through tissue areas that are not the intended target. Two examples where the desired effect on tissue is of the transmission type are in the treatment of bladder tumors and the coagulation of the blood vessels on the retina.

Absorption of the laser beam occurs when the tissue takes the wavelength into its surface and sublayers. Tissue damage occurs as the tissue absorbs the laser energy and produces heat. The cellular water is superheated to over 100° C, causing intracellular protein to be destroyed. The water inside the cell turns to steam, and as the cellular membrane ruptures, debris and smoke, commonly called laser plume, are expelled from the tissue. The depth of penetration of the laser beam and the thermal destruction of the tissue are influenced by several variables. They include wavelength, power density, fluence of the beam, duration of the beam, color, consistency, and water content of the tissue. These factors determine the appropriate settings and types of lasers to be used for surgical cases.

Tissue response can be thermal, mechanical, or chemical. About 85% of all lasers used today produce a thermal effect at the tissue level. The lasers in this category can cut, coagulate, seal, weld tissue, vaporize, and ablate tissue. Some lasers produce mechanical effects on tissue by generating sonic energy that mechanically disrupts tissue. Other lasers produce a chemical effect when the laser energy activates light-sensitive drugs to destroy malignant cells [4].

Benefits of Laser Surgery

Benefits to laser surgery can be viewed from three different perspectives. First is the patient. Some of the positive results of laser surgery for the patient are reduced pain and edema following surgery. The laser also can provide excellent hemostasis, minimal damage to contiguous tissue, automatic sealing of lymphatics, and minimal scar formation. All of these factors can make the postoperative recovery period shorter and less stressful.

The physician also can see positive benefits when using the laser. It has pinpoint accuracy with a touch or nontouch technique. The laser is also readily adaptable to different surgical procedures and easy to control. The surgery is highly sterile because of the beam, which allows the field to be dry, thus reducing blood transfusions. Surgeons now can perform surgery that was not possible by other methods and provide better patient care because of the laser's vast potential.

The institution also benefits from lasers. It is an advanced technology that can improve the image of the hospital from the patients' and surgeons' perspectives. If a surgeon/patient has a preference for using a specific laser for a procedure, it allows the surgery to be performed. It also can impact length of stay for patients, reduce cost, and possibly provide services not previously available in the community.

LASER SYSTEMS

Each laser is identified by its wavelength and lasing medium. Because each lasing medium produces one wavelength and one frequency range, each will have a different effect on tissue.

Carbon Dioxide Laser

There are two types of CO_2 laser, the free-flowing and the sealed tube; both types use a gas medium. The free-flowing CO_2 laser uses gas cylinders containing a special mixture of CO_2, nitrogen, and helium. The laser beam is created by an exact mixture of the three gases. A vacuum pump is also necessary to create the subatmospheric pressure needed in the laser tube during the lasing period. The gas cylinders need to be monitored and changed when empty. All of these components add to the cost, noise, and maintenance of this laser. The sealed tube laser system contains a special mixture of CO_2, nitrogen, helium, and several other gases sealed within the laser tube. Sealed tube lasers have an operating and a shelf life. The operating life refers to the laser unit, while the shelf life refers to the expected life of the sealed laser tube before it needs recharging. This time frame depends on the technology used in the manufacturing of the tube and ranges from 1 to 4 years. The cost to recharge the tube can be nominal or quite expensive. This factor needs to be considered when deciding which type of CO_2 laser is best for the institution. Because the sealed tube technology uses radio frequency or electrical current to excite the CO_2, a vacuum pump and replacement gas cylinders are not needed for its operation. These systems produce less noise and are mechanically and electronically simpler to operate [4].

The wavelength of the CO_2 laser is 10,600 nm, and it located in the middle infrared region of the electromagnetic spectrum. This wavelength is invisible; therefore it requires an additional visible laser beam to be present during its operation. Because the wavelength is long, the beam is delivered through a hollow tube with mirrors positioned at the joints. This hollow tube is referred to as the articulating arm. The mirrors, which are reflective and partially reflective, allow the invisible CO_2 beam and the visible red helium–neon (HeNe) beam, referred to as the aiming beam, to be moved forward in the tube. Misalignment of the articulating arm can cause these beams to be projected on the tissue at different places, causing serious problems or injuries to delicate tissues when fired.

There are various lens devices that can be attached to the end of the articulating arm, causing the raw laser beam to be concentrated into a small spot, called the focal point of the beam. A lens always needs to be positioned in front of the raw laser beam, or a potential safety hazard can occur, since the raw beam is able to travel great distances. A hand piece with a lens can be attached to the articulating arm of the laser, allowing the surgeon to use the laser in a freehand mode. The articulating arm of the CO_2 laser can be adapted to a microscope or colposcope. The focal length of the microscope/colposcope must be coordinated with the focal length of the laser lens. Also, the beam can be delivered to the tissue by connecting the articulating arm to a coupling device that then is attached to a rigid endoscope. CO_2 laser lenses need to be handled with care and cannot be soaked or autoclaved because of their specialty coating. This coating of zinc selenide or gallium arsenide provides for the antireflection of the beam to ensure that both the HeNe and CO_2 beams are approximately the same size.

The depth of penetration (0.05 mm) of the CO_2 beam is controlled by the power density and the duration of exposure to the beam. When a cutting mode is desired, the laser needs to be at a higher power within a smaller focused beam and with a shorter exposure time to decrease the spread of thermal energy to adjacent tissue. If coagulation is desired, the beam needs to be defocused to enlarge the spot size and spread the energy over a larger area. The beam will continue to travel after it cuts or coagulates tissue; therefore, a backstop is needed to decrease the damage to adjacent tissue. This can be accomplished with a wet sponge or rods made of quartz or titanium.

The CO_2 laser system has various modes that can be selected and used during use. They have different functions and tissue interaction. The continuous wave (CW) allows the beam to continuously hit the tissue while the foot pedal is depressed. The single pulse mode delivers a single pulse of the chosen wattage for a specified time. The time that is chosen needs to programmed into the settings. The repeat pulse or time mode allows the beam to hit the tissue at a particular wattage and for a specified time as long as the foot pedal is being depressed. This time period must be programmed into the unit before starting. The superpulse mode is a beam that is turning on and off at a tremendously fast rate. This mode allows the tissue to cool, thus resulting in less damage to adjacent tissue. This mode is used when precision is critical. The physician will chose the mode that will achieve the desired effect on the tissue for each particular case.

Neodymium: Yttrium Aluminum Garnet Laser

The Nd:YAG laser uses a crystal medium of yttrium, aluminum, and garnet. It is doped or laced with a rare element called neodymium. Its laser energy is produced when electrical current passes through the optical power source of bright flash lamps. Because a great amount of heat is generated by this modality, air, carbon dioxide, or water is needed as a cooling system.

The wavelength of the Nd:YAG laser is 1064 nm, in the near-infrared region of the electromagnetic spectrum. Because this wavelength is invisible, it also requires a visible aiming beam when used. Usually a red HeNe beam is used in conjunction with this laser, but other blue or white lights can be used as the aiming beam. This laser beam can be delivered to tissue by means of a contact or noncontact fiber delivery system.

The noncontact fiber delivery system uses a quartz fiber, and the laser light is introduced into the fiber by a lens system at its proximal end. The laser beam traverses the length of the fiber by a process called total internal reflection. The fiberoptic of the fiber is made up of a core and its cladding, which provides flexibility and stability to the fiber. This composite allows the fiber to easily bend without compromising the delivery of the laser energy. Usually this type of fiber is called a bare or straight fiber. A catheter fiber is surrounded by a sheath that permits purge air, gas, or fluid to flow along its length to cool its distal end. When the Nd:YAG laser first was introduced, reusable fibers were the only type of fibers available. Fibers needed to be stripped, cleaved, calibrated, and autoclaved after every use according to the manufacturer's instructions. This is time-consuming, and usually only selected personnel were trained to perform this task.

With the development of a contact fiber delivery system, the surgeon regained tactile sensation during surgery. Special ceramic or sapphire tips are used for this system. As the name suggests, the fiber's beam now can come in direct contact with the intended tissue. Cutting and vaporization can be achieved without diffuse coagulation. These tips can be used freehand like a scalpel or be fitted on the end of fiber for use with an endoscope. Because these tips have a high temperature threshold, low heat conductivity, and are very strong, they can be reused if properly handled, cleaned, and autoclaved. Single-use fibers with tips are available and replaced the reusable fibers. In today's market, however, cost containment strategies of reusing fibers are being evaluated for potential cost savings.

When the noncontact fiber's energy impacts tissue, it has a high degree of scattering, with thermal damage occurring to a depth of 5 mm. The beam is absorbed poorly in water and hemoglobin but highly absorbed by tissue protein. Because of this property, this laser has the most powerful coagulation capability of any surgical laser. The Nd:YAG laser is used in the CW mode. As the beam continues to coagulate, it progresses to vaporization. Carbonization is the by-product of this vaporization, and it makes the tissue absorb the beam more readily. This leads to greater tissue absorption, reaction, and plume formation. The contact tip has a lesser degree of scattering, because the tip is in actual contact with the tissue, allowing for greater precision, less adjacent thermal tissue damage, and less production of plume.

The Nd:YAG laser is used in the CW mode. These systems may have special electrical requirements and also may require special plugs dedicated to the laser. Water-cooled units require external plumbing hookups to keep the laser head cooled. Adequate water flow is essential for the laser to function. Other laser systems are air-cooled, with a contained internal water supply cooled by a fan system. Besides the CW mode, a special Nd:YAG laser was developed that delivered energy in a pulse mode. This modality delivers energy to the tissue in nanoseconds and is used in ophthalmology. The Q-switched Nd:YAG is another laser that delivers power in tens of nanoseconds. Because the pulses are of short duration, it does not have a thermal effect on tissue. This laser does not have any special electrical or water requirements [4].

Holmium: Yttrium-Aluminum-Garnet Lasers

The holmium: yttrium-aluminum-garnet (Ho:YAG) laser uses a crystal yttrium-aluminum-garnet that is doped with holmium, thulium, and chromium. These elements increase the wavelength to 2100 nm, in the midinfrared range of the electromagnetic spectrum. This invisible wavelength also needs a red HeNe aiming beam to be added to the laser. The excitation medium of this laser is flash lamps that pass through a solid rod of holmium that has curved mirrors attached at either end of the rod. An external water hook-up is not needed, because it is cooled internally.

This wavelength is delivered to the tissue in a quick pulsed mode readily absorbed by water. Because the beam is not color-selective, its depth of penetration is limited to 0.4 to 0.6 mm, similar to the CO_2 laser beam. This beam can be delivered to tissue by a flexible fiber and in a fluid environment. When used in a fluid medium, the beam produces a vapor bubble that transmits the energy to the tissue but does not produce char or extensive tissue damage. If the fiber is touching or held closely to the tissue, it will cut. Holding the fiber approximately 2 mm from the target tissue will allow the surgeon to sculpt or ablate tissue. No tissue response will be noted if the fiber is held 5 mm from the target tissue. This laser also can be used to produce a photo–acoustical effect that is useful when fragmenting urinary and gall stones [5].

Erbium: Yttrium-Aluminum-Garnet Lasers

The erbium: yttrium-aluminum-garnet (Er:YAG) laser is a solid crystal laser that generates a wavelength of 2940 nm. This laser also uses a visible secondary beam during its use, because it is in the infrared range of the electromagnetic spectrum. Like the Ho:YAG, the laser energy delivered to the tissue is in a pulsed modality. At low pulse energy, surgery on very fine tissue structures like the ear can be accomplished. This wavelength also is absorbed well in water, allowing for shallow penetration of the beam. The surrounding tissue is barely injured. This laser is one of the most recent to be introduced into health care [5].

Potassium Titanyl Phosphate Lasers

The potassium titanyl phosphate (KPT) laser uses a crystal medium of potassium titanyl and phosphate. To produce its beam, an Nd:YAG incident beam of 1064 nm is passed through the potassium titanyl phosphate crystal. The resulting emergent beam is a visible shortened 532 nm beam that is bright green in color. When the beam is shortened, the frequency of the beam is doubled. The system has the ability to allow the user to select the incident Nd:YAG beam or the emergent KTP beam by switching a button on the console, it is called a frequency doubled YAG laser. The KTP beam is transmitted through clear fluids and structures but is absorbed by hemoglobin, melanin, and other similar pigments [4].

This laser also has special electrical and water requirements. If the water temperature or pressure is too low to cool the unit, special safety features will prohibit the laser from firing. Error codes displayed on the console will alert the user to this problem.

The laser delivery system can be delivered through a fiber or a microscope. If using a microscope, a special eye filter is adapted to the scope. During surgery, the surgeon has a clear field until the laser is activated. Upon firing the laser, the filter drops into place to protect the surgeon's eyes from damage. The fiber delivery system is made up of a quartz core surrounded by cladding and nylon coating to protect it from breakage. These fibers can be reused, but they need to be calibrated and processed according to the manufacturer's directions. Also, the fiber can be used for either wavelength, 1064 or 532 nm, and in the contact or noncontact mode.

Argon Lasers

The argon laser produces beams whose wavelengths are 488 and 514.5 nm, respectively. On the electromagnetic spectrum, these wavelengths are visible and are an intense blue and green color. The plasma tube, containing the argon, is the core of the system and requires a high electrical current to be passed down the tube to excite the argon ions to produce laser energy. Although the argon laser has become more reliable, the cost to replace the plasma tube can be expensive.

The argon laser energy passes through clear fluids and structures, but this wavelength selectively and readily absorbs hemoglobin, melanin, or other similar pigmentation. Its depth of penetration is 1 or 2 mm in most tissue. Because the argon beam is visible, it technically does not require an aiming beam to see its wavelength. To prevent injury or damage to other structures, however, this laser uses a low-power energy beam to indicate where the high-power beam will strike. Usually alignment of the two laser beams is not an issue or problem.

The argon laser uses an electrical power source and internal fans to cool the unit, but in higher power units the electrical requirements increase along with an external water supply to cool the tube. To meet these increased demands to the unit, a booster pump can be added.

The argon delivery system can be through a slit lamp or microscope. When using this modality, an internal optical filter is used to protect the surgeon's eyes during the firing of the laser. Also, a flexible fiber can be used to deliver the laser beam to the tissue. The fiber can be passed through a biopsy port of a rigid or semirigid endoscope. Usually, these fibers are used in a noncontact mode, but some fibers can be used by touching the tissue. Also, a fiber can be encapsulated in a cannula for use in the eyes or ears; it is usually disposable. A hand piece, attached to a fiber, can be used to alter the laser beam [4].

Tunable Dye Lasers

This laser has a limited wavelength range of 400 to 1000 nm, in the visible range of the electromagnetic spectrum. The variable wave length is achieved by dissolving liquid organic dye in a suitable medium and then exposing it to an intense light source. The dye absorbs the laser light, then fluoresces and emits light over a board spectrum of visible color. A specific wavelength is obtained by turning a special element, such as a birefringent filter, through various angles on the console. The tuneable dye laser also is used in photodynamic therapy. Tunable dye lasers can be used in the continuous or pulsed mode, but they have been refined to provide pulsations in milliseconds. Scanners using this quick pulsation have been developed. Attachment to the delivery system allows movement of the beam over the target area with less adjacent tissue injury [4].

Excimer Lasers

The wavelengths of the excimer laser are located in the ultraviolet range of the electromagnetic spectrum. Originally, this laser's active medium was an excited dimer, which refers to a molecule that is relatively stable when excited. Today, the excimer laser system uses an excited complex of rare gases and halogen but retains the same name. The chemical composition of the active medium produces the exact wavelength, and several popular gases are used today in excimer lasers. The four most popular ultraviolet wavelengths produced from gas are: xenon fluoride (XeF) at 351 nm, xenon chloride (XeCl) at 308 nm, krypton fluoride (KrF), and argon fluoride (ArF) at 193 nm. One of the hazards of these lasers is the toxicity of the gases used to produce their wavelength. Their use in clinical practice will continue to grow as long as appropriate measures are taken to make them safe. The excimer laser has significant photo ablation ability. The depth of penetration of the beam is less than 1 mm. It disassociates the molecular bonds of the cells without producing thermal energy. A sharp clean cut is produced at the target site without damage to the adjacent tissues [5].

Diode Lasers

Diode lasers are compact efficient lasers primarily used in consumer products such as computers, fiberoptic communication, video disc players, and assorted electronic instruments and equipment. In surgical lasers, the wavelengths are in the 750 to 950 nm range. One such laser is the smaller high-powered semiconductor diode laser in the gallium arsenide family whose wavelength is in the 840 to 910 nm range. The laser energy from this range can be delivered directly to tissue by a fiber or by attaching it to a slit-lamp microscope [5].

LASER SAFETY

Because the laser has the ability to concentrate tremendous amounts of power into a small spot, the potential dangers of the laser are apparent. It is imperative that the surgical team understand each laser's wavelength and the safety precautions that are required to protect the patient and staff from any hazards that may occur during the use of lasers during surgery.

Laser Regulatory Bodies and Classifications

Several federal regulatory bodies and nongovernmental agencies have developed regulations or guidelines for the safe use of lasers. The Center for

Devices & Radiological Health (CDRH) is the regulatory section of the US Food and Drug Administration (FDA), and it is responsible for standardizing the manufacturing of laser units. This agency is also responsible for the specific labeling that is required on all class IV lasers. The Occupational Safety & Health Administration (OSHA) is within the US Department of Labor, and it is responsible for the safety of the worker during laser use. The American National Standards Institute (ANSI) is a voluntary agency composed of experts from different fields who developed standards for the safe use of lasers. This agency is considered the authority on lasers, and existing federal and state safety regulations concerning lasers are based on its standards. The Association of Operating Room Nurses (AORN) is a professional nursing organization that has developed standards for the safe use of lasers by the perioperative nurse. These standards are considered to be the optimal level of practice for nurses involved with lasers. Although state and local regulations concerning the laser may vary from area to area, every health care facility that uses surgical lasers must have standards or protocols in place that address protective measures for the safe use of lasers, education of the users, the laser safety officer (LSO), and management of accidents.

Because the laser is a medical device, it falls under the jurisdiction of the medical device regulations published in 1975. The laser is classified as a class 3 medical device that is subdivided into four more divisions. Class I refers to items that are self-contained and used in laboratories for diagnostic work. This group usually does not inflict harm under normal circumstances and is subject to general controls. In class II, the devices could cause harm if viewed for extended periods of time, such as a HeNe laser pointer, and general controls are not sufficient. Class III devices require special training to operate and have a high potential for injury. The surveyor lasers are an example and these lasers that require procedural controls and protective equipment. Class IV lasers are classified as potentially hazardous, and they could cause fires, skin burns, and retinal damage either by direct or indirect reflective contact. Most lasers used in the hospital setting are class IV and require strict safety protocols.

Although many agencies contribute to the regulations/standards of safe laser use, each health care facility must address laser safety in its own environment. The institution can oversee the use of the lasers in by using an LSO, the laser committee, and laser nurse specialists. The LSO has an in-depth knowledge and training in the use of lasers and is responsible for overseeing the safe practice of laser use in the institution. The laser committee monitors and ensures laser safety within the institution and works closely with the LSO. One of its most important functions is developing and monitoring credentialing protocols for surgeons who want to use the laser. Credentialing is the formal recognition by the hospital of a surgeon's ability to perform a specific surgical operation and the granting of permission by a hospital to do so on its premises [6]. Another function of this committee is to develop policies and procedures for the safe use of lasers, and the committee has the authority to enforce these standards. Laser nurse specialists are members of the staff who are trained specifically in the use of lasers. They are usually under the direction of the LSO. As laser use continues to evolve, health care must not only met today's standards for a safe environment for patient and staff but must look toward the future.

Patient Safety

During any surgical intervention, patient safety is one of the surgical team's primary concerns and functions. This is even more important when surgery involves the use of a laser. To protect the patient from injury, the team needs to have in-depth knowledge of the safety standards and protocols in place for that laser. During the preoperative assessment, the circulating nurse should explain any safety intervention that may require the patient's participation (eg, wearing of protective eyewear and wearing a high filtration mask). One of the greatest concerns during the use of the laser is protection of the patient's eyes. This is the responsibility of the anesthesia and operating room teams. When the patient is awake or sedated, the appropriate eyewear must be worn by the patient. If the patient is under general anesthesia, moistened eye pads should be taped over the eyes. If using the Nd:YAG, a laser-retardant drape should be placed over the eyes, because moistened pads will not inhibit this beam. If the laser is being used on the eyelid or in the immediate vicinity, metal eye shields are available. Care must be taken not to injure the eye.

The next area of concern is the prepping solution that will be used. Ideally this solution should be a nonflammable skin preparation, and the perioperative staff should ensure that no fluid pool on or around the skin [7]. If prep pads were used, they should be removed and the skin allowed to dry.

At the surgical site, the immediate area around the incision should be protected from thermal damage. Flammable material in the area needs to be restricted. Moisten towels are placed around the surgical field to prevent accidental ignition of the surgical drapes. Sponges, towels, or surgical patties always should be moistened when placed near or around the target tissue. If using the Nd:YAG, however, these items need to be removed from the area, because wetting does not prohibit the beam from penetrating them. When involved with perineal cases, the rectum should be packed with a moistened sponge to prevent the escape of methane gas from the intestinal tract. This gas can ignite an explosion. Care also must be taken with the laser hand piece; it should be monitored and placed in a secure area when not in use.

Anesthetic agents should be noncombustible and when mixed with oxygen should be delivered in a closed system. If lasing during oral, laryngeal, bronchial, or esophageal procedures and using nitrous oxide and oxygen, the concentration should be as low as possible around the head. Laser-approved endotracheal tubes are available for aerodigestive cases. The endotracheal tube should be inflated with normal saline solution, and to detect a leak in the cuff, the solution can be tinged with methylene blue. Unprotected polyvinyl chloride (PVC) endotracheal tubes can be ignited by a laser beam and will emit offensive hydrogen chloride fumes. Airway fires are life-threatening for the patient and require immediate intervention by the team.

Another area of concern for the patient is the plume. If the patient is awake or sedated during the use of the CO_2 laser for ablation cases, such as condylomas, the patient should wear a high filtration mask for protection from inhaling airborne material into the lungs. Intubated patients are not considered at risk for respiratory contamination.

Personnel Safety

Eye safety is one of the most critical elements to be addressed in any laser case, because the eyes are susceptible to laser radiation. Eye protection is necessary for all personnel in the room. The exact portion of the eye at risk for injury varies with the wavelength of the laser in use. Wavelengths in the ultraviolet (200 to 400 nm), midinfrared (1400 to 3000 nm), and far infrared (3000 to 10,600 nm) spectrum primarily are absorbed by the cornea and lens. The near infrared (760 to 1400 nm) and visible (400 to 760 nm) wavelength primarily are absorbed by the retina and vascular choroid of the eye [8]. These injuries would be the same for the patient, but their exposure to the laser is not as frequent as the staff's exposure. Recommended standards suggest that all laser eyewear be inscribed with its optical density, which is the ability of the lens to absorb a specific wavelength. The correct optical density eyewear needs to be worn by all personnel during the use of the laser. Protective eyewear must shield the eyes from the top, bottom and sides of the visual field and should transmit as much visible light as possible. Color distortion may occur with protective eyewear used with wavelengths in the visible and near infrared range. Contact lenses, half glasses and user's prescription lenses are not considered appropriate eyewear and will not protect the wearer against eye injury. Microscopes or endoscopes use protective filters or lenses to protect the user from eye injury, because the required glasses/goggles may interfere with the surgeon's vision. If multiple wavelengths are being used during a case, the eyewear needs to match the wavelength and may need to be changed on patient and personnel. Although certain eyewear can have a certain range and provide protection for several different wavelengths, there is no eyewear on the market that protects the eye from all the possible wavelengths. Because protective eyewear can be expensive, it must be handled properly and appropriately stored to prevent any type of damage to the lenses or frames. Some institutions provide a baseline eye examination for employees who routinely are exposed to the laser, but performing eye examinations has nothing to do with guaranteeing eye safety.

Laser plume, which is the result of vaporization of the tissue during laser ablation, contains water, carbonized particles, mutated DNA cells, and intact cells. Vaporization of only 1 g of tissue has been shown to be the same as smoking six unfiltered cigarettes and creates smoke that is 52% more concentrated than government standards allow. Small exposures during a period of years can lead to airway narrowing or emphysema [9]. To prevent the inhalation of these fumes, a smoke evacuation system with a charcoal filter should be used. The charcoal filter will reduce odor and trap the toxic flumes. Because the particle matter in the plume may be less than 1.1 μg, a high filtration mask should be worn by all personnel in the room. Smoke evacuation from the surgical site helps improve visibility and also diminishes the chance that the laser beam could be bent or refracted. If using a suction system, there should be an in-line filter to protect the wall suction. The suction canister and in-line filters should be changed after every case. Gloves and masks should be worn when handling these contaminated items. Commercial smoke evacuators usually have a charcoal filter and need to be changed according to the manufacturer's instructions.

The area where the laser is being used needs to be controlled by the laser team members. This area needs to have restricted traffic, and personnel entering the area should be trained in laser safety. If there are any windows or ports in the room, they need to be covered with a barrier that does not allow the laser beam to penetrate the room. Laser signs need to be posted at every entrance to the room. The signs will state the laser's classification, hazard symbol, the word DANGER written at the top with LASER RADIATION warning, and the appropriate eyewear that is required. It may be easier to enforce eye safety during the case if the appropriate glasses/goggles are hung near the sign. Some laser signs can be turned around to let the staff know that the laser is not being used at a particular time, and personnel may enter without eye protection. Laser signs need to be removed when the case if finished.

Door interlock systems also can be installed on laser systems. This device automatically prevents the laser from being fired or shuts down the laser during use if the door is opened. This safety feature can be a potential hazard to the patient if the physician is coagulating bleeders or is at a critical stage of dissection.

The laser needs to be checked and tested before the patient is brought into the operating room. A checklist can be used for each type of laser. Any malfunctions need to be documented and resolved before the laser can be used. The laser keys should be stored in a safe place, and only personnel with appropriate training should have access to them. During the procedure, there should be direct communication between the surgeon and the laser operator, and all commands should be repeated for accuracy. When the laser is not in use, it should be in standby mode. The laser never should be on and left unattended. The surgeon delivering the laser energy should give the laser commands and operate the laser foot pedal. All other foot pedals should be removed from the surgeon to diminish the chance of an accidental firing of the laser. Nonreflective instruments should be used during laser surgery to prevent burns or fires from reflective surfaces. These instruments can be a dull blue titanium alloy, coated, ebonized, or anodized stainless steel.

All lasers have electrical requirements to operate. Some have special electrical plugs/outlets, while others can be plugged into the receptacle located in the room. Whatever the requirement, care must be taken to avoid electrical hazards that may present during surgery. All staff should know the location of circuit breakers within the suite. Also, any specific requirements will be listed in the manufacturer's guide. This guide additionally will give instructions on use, care, and handling of the laser and any accessory equipment.

Fire is another potential hazard that can occur when using a laser. All personnel should be aware of the protocol to follow in the event of a fire. A basin of sterile water or normal saline solution should be on the field and available for immediate use, because drapes that consist of cloth are highly combustible. Towels that are saturated with water or normal saline decrease their flammable properties but need to be monitored constantly and periodically moistened. Disposable drapes, however, generally are treated with a flame-retardant substance and once ignited are difficult to extinguish [10]. Because water is repelled with these drapes, an appropriate fire extinguisher needs to be readily available. Because fire needs oxygen to burn, the oxygen concentration in the room should be as low as possible. Leakage from a loose-fitting face mask could be a potential hazard if the laser beam is being used in the vicinity. During the course of the case, never place any type of liquid on the laser or smoke evacuator units. If any fluid is spilled and gets into the unit, it could act as a conductor and short-circuit the units. A halon fire extinguisher should be available in the room by the laser in event of the laser unit catching fire. This extinguisher disrupts combustion by interrupting the flaming process and does not produce a residue. There are environmental concerns, however, because the halon disrupts the ozone layer of the earth's atmosphere.

CLINICAL LASER APPLICATIONS

Laser technology has evolved over the years and now is available for use in many specialties. As new wavelengths continue to be developed or perfected for clinical use, their applications in surgery become limitless.

Ophthalmology

Ophthalmologists have been the forerunners in using the laser. Many procedures can be performed in the office or as an outpatient using little or no anesthesia. Routinely, the argon laser is used for retinal photocoagulation. The energy from this laser can be delivered through the clear structures of the eye to one spot or around the retina to seal new blood vessels. The retinal pigmentation's hemoglobin and melania are absorbed by the blue-green beam of this laser. To help prevent macular damage, a filter may be used to deliver only the green beam to the target area, and many physicians prefer using only the green beam. Tunable dye yellow laser and the frequency doubled Nd:YAG also may be used to threat this condition. In the last few years, however, the diode laser has become the laser of choice for photocoagulation, because it is compact, reliable, and easy to move and maintain. Another use for the argon and diode lasers is in the treatment of retinal tears and detachments. Laser energy is delivered to the area of the tear by an intraocular probe or through a slit lamp. Placements of photocoagulated sealing spots around the tears causes an adhesive scar. This scar formation stops the progression of the tear, thus preventing a detachment [4].

The argon or Nd:YAG lasers are used to treat open-angle glaucoma. The argon beam is directed through a three-mirrored contact lens. It then forms photocoagulated spots along the pigmented zone of the midtrabecular meshwork, while the Nd:YAG laser beam produces holes along the trabecular network. With either laser therapy, topical and systemic medications are continued after the procedure to ensure decreased intraocular pressure. If the pressure rises again, repeat laser therapy may be required. To treat close-angle glaucoma, an iridectomy is performed. This can be accomplished with an argon or Nd:YAG laser. The iridectomy allows the aqueous humor to flow from the posterior chamber into the anterior chamber. Both laser beams use short-duration pulses to make a small hole in the iris.

The excimer laser is used for keratorefractive procedures on the cornea. The wavelength of this laser's beam is ideal for use on the cornea, because it has no significant thermal buildup and is so precise in it delivery that it only affects one cell at a time. Photorefractive keratectomy (PRK) uses the argon fluoride (ArF) excimer laser to ablate the central portion of the cornea to treat myopia or nearsightedness. Laser-assisted in situ keratomileusis, commonly referred to as LASIK, uses the excimer laser to treat both myopia and hyperopia, commonly called farsightedness. In the treatment of hyperopia, the cornea needs to be made steeper. This is achieved by removing the stromal tissue from the periphery of the cornea while leaving the center portion of the cornea unchanged [5].

Other lasers being used in ophthalmology are the Er:YAG laser to perform anterior capsulotomy during cataract extraction, or the Ho:YAG laser for sclerostomy, used to treat glaucoma and also for corneal sculpting.

Neurosurgery

The CO_2 laser was the first laser used by the neurosurgeons because of its ability for precise dissection and hemostasis. These qualities make the resection of brain tumors less traumatic for the patient and easier to accomplish for the surgeon. With controlled hemostasis, the surgical field stays drier, which leads to greater visual acuity for the surgeon and less blood loss for the patient. Removal of brain tumors can be accomplished with the CO_2, KTP, or contact Nd:YAG lasers. The contact Nd:YAG laser has several distinct advantages over the other wavelengths for excision of brain lesions. The advantages are: no carbonization of the edges of the tissue, minimal plume formation, control of the dissecting plane (because it is now a touching modality), and greater access to deeper tumor tissue. The lasers also can be used in stereotactic endoscopic brain surgery. When using contact fibers with detachable tips, the junction must be cooled with coaxial gas or fluid. For open procedures, air or CO_2 coolant is a sufficient medium. Do not use air, or any other gas, as a coaxial fiber coolant of the probe in areas where the risk of air embolism exists. The contact Nd:YAG laser also is being used to remove spinal cord tumors. This has been made easier with the development of spinal endoscopes that provide direct visualization of spine. Vascular lesions of the brain are being treated with argon and double frequency YAG lasers. Because these wavelengths are color-selective, the pigmentation in the tumor absorbs the laser energy, while the surrounding tissue is unharmed. KTP lasers also are used in microvascular surgery; they are especially useful when sealing vessels less than 0.5mm in diameter [11].

Podiatry

The most commonly used laser of the podiatrist is the CO_2. This laser is used to treat certain nail conditions. A laser matrixectomy, either partial or total, treats ingrown nails by ablating the matrix tissue where nail growth is not desired. Sixty percent of people over the age of fifty have onychomycosis or fungus nail. This condition is treated by vaporizing the fungal spores but preserving the matrix of the nail. Subungual hematomas are treated by burning five to six holes into the nail plate without anesthesia. Morton's neuroma can be excised with a CO_2 or contact Nd:YAG laser. Although heel spurs can be treated with these lasers, it may not be cost-effective [4].

Orthopedic

The CO_2 laser was the first wavelength to gain acceptance for use in arthroscopy of the knee. This wavelength could not be used in a fluid medium, so a gas medium was required. Because formation of an air embolus was a real concern, a tourniquet was used routinely during the procedure. The contact Nd:YAG laser also can be used in arthroscopies. The advantages are: its energy can be delivered through a fluid medium; depth of penetration is controlled, and there is decreased damage to the surrounding tissue. Today, the most commonly used laser for arthroscopies of the knee, shoulder, or ankle is the Ho:YAG. Its energy is delivered to the target tissue in a fluid medium through the arthroscope or a secondary puncture site by means of a flexible fiber. The advantage of this laser is the beam's precise ablation and shallow depth of penetration.

The KTP and Ho:YAG are used for laser discectomy to ablate the center of the herniated disc to relieve leg pain. This procedure can be done percutaneously or through a small incision. Direct visualization is facilitated by the use of spinal endoscopes. The pulsed laser beam's shallow penetration ablates the nucleus without damaging the nerve root, and local anesthesia is used, so the patient can communicate any pain in a particular area during the procedure. The patient is discharged the same day, because this procedure is considered minimally invasive [4].

In total joint arthroplasty, a bone cement called polymethyl methacrylate (PMMA) can be used to stabilize the joint components. If there is a failure, a revision procedure is performed, and the surgeon is faced with the task of removing the PMMA during the case. The CO_2 laser beam can cut and vaporize the PMMA easily. The plume's by-products, including methyl methacrylate, formalin, acetylene, benzene, carbon monoxide and other trace gases, need to be removed by a high-power smoke evacuation system to protect patient and staff [12].

During soft tissue dissection, the CO_2, contact Nd:YAG, Ho:YAG, and KTP lasers can ablate and vaporize adipose tissue, fascia, and muscle. The laser can replace the electrocautery as a dissection tool during surgery, and it also can coagulate bleeding vessels.

Laser biostimulation uses a HeNe laser beam. This cold laser treatment is a nonsurgical intervention used to decrease pain in joints or pain from previous surgeries. Usually this is done as a series of treatments, but more research is being done in this area to prove the laser's efficacy.

Peripheral Vascular/Cardiothoracic

There are various treatment options for patients with advanced arteriosclerosis that is compromising tissue profusion. One such treatment option is balloon angioplasty with the laser. The laser destroys the plaque, while the balloon increases the channel of the vessel for blood flow. Laser angioplasty can be achieved by thermal, photothermal, or photochemical therapy. In thermal laser angioplasty, the argon or Nd:YAG laser beams are used to heat a tip attached to a fiberoptic waveguide within the plaque in the vessel. High temperatures created inside the vessel can cause carbonization and necrosis of the vessel layers. With photothermal laser angioplasty, the plaque is heated to the point of vaporization using a contact Nd:YAG probe. Decreased arterial injury is noted with this method. Photochemical laser angioplasty originally used the excimer laser with different combinations of gases to generate its various wavelengths. It ablates by breaking the bonds of the plaque with sock waves. No carbonization is formed, leaving the vessel's intima smooth. Serious safety concerns, however, center on using this laser because of its possible disruption of DNA and the highly toxic nature of the gases being used. These concerns have led to research in using the Ho:YAG. This laser energy also can break the bonds of the plaque without any of the safety concerns mentioned [4]. Laser angioplasty can be performed by a radiologist, cardiologist, or surgeon. The setting for the procedure usually is scheduled where the specialist performs most of his or her work.

With successful peripheral laser angioplasty being performed, the development of coronary laser angioplasty soon followed. In this procedure, plaque is destroyed selectively by introducing a small flexible fiber to the blockage. This intervention has potential complications such as perforation, vessel spasms, cardiac arrhythmia, intimal dissection, and reocclusion. Because coronary artery disease affects so many people, however, this treatment modality will continue to be refined and grow.

Transmyocardial revascularization is performed to increase inadequate perfusion of the heart. A CO_2 or Ho:YAG laser beam drills small holes into the heart's left ventricle. This is done in a region of the myocardium where reversible ischemia is present but is not amenable to revascularization by direct coronary artery grafting.

Laser-assisted vascular anastomosis, also referred to as vascular tissue welding, fuses 6 to 8 mm-sized vessels together using an argon laser. The anastomosis is performed using an operating microscope. This anastomosis also can be used to create an arteriovenous shunt for hemodialysis, to reattach severed limbs, and to repair damaged vessels [11].

In thoracic surgery, the CO_2 or Nd:YAG laser is used for treating tracheo–bronchial lesions through a bronchoscope. Malignant or benign lesions of the mainstem bronchus and trachea that are obstructive also can be treated with this laser therapy. During thoracoscopy, the Nd:YAG laser can be used to treat bullous emphysema, which affects a large numbers of smokers or former smokers.

Plastic Surgery and Dermatology

Many conditions can be treated by dermatologists and plastic surgeons in their office or in an outpatient surgery center. The yellow light and argon lasers are effective in treating port wine stains and hemangiomas. Spider veins, especially on the legs, are responding to the yellow light laser. Scars and keloids are being removed with CO_2, Nd:YAG, argon, and yellow light lasers. The CO_2 laser is used for dermabrasion to treat psoriasis, acne, and wrinkles. The contact Nd:YAG and CO_2 lasers also are used to treat warts. The CO_2, argon, pulsed ruby, and Nd:YAG lasers have been used to remove decorative tattoo pigmentation from the skin. The CO_2 laser energy is used in the removal of cosmetic tattoos, laser blepharoplasty, and in repairing pierced ear trauma [4].

In reduction mammoplasty, the excess skin and glandular tissue may be excised with a CO_2 laser. Because breast tissue is very vascular, hemostasis is critical. The advantage of using the CO_2 laser is the ability of the beam to coagulate small blood vessels and seal the lymphatics as the tissue is excised.

Otorhinolaryngology

Otolaryngologists began using the laser in 1967 when it was adapted for use on the microscope. Endoscopic treatment of many benign and malignant lesions of the larynx is facilitated by the use of the laser. The CO_2 laser is the most commonly used wavelength for laser microlaryngoscopy. The CO_2 microslad is attached to the microscope, and the laser beam is manipulated with a joy stick to the target area. Teeth need to be protected from injury and from accidental beam impact, but the biggest safety issue during this procedure is an airway fire. Special endotracheal (ET) tubes are used to protect the airway and never should be taped in place. Small counted cottonoid sponges are soaked in saline and placed around the ET tube with their strings placed away from the laser's path. During the case, the sponges are monitored constantly and moistened if needed. If airway combustion occurs, all gases are stopped; the ignited ET tube is removed, and oxygen is administered. Bronchoscopy equipment should be immediately available. The patient may be reintubated with a smaller ET tube. A tracheostomy may be necessary to ventilate the patient. Further treatment is dictated by the extent of the injury. All members of the team should know the protocol for action in the event of an airway fire. The immediate response and actions of the team can impact the patient's outcome. Another safety issue is the removal of the plume. Visual acuity is hampered by the smoke, and inhalation of the plume by the patient could be hazardous. A smoke evacuator is essential for the safe removal of the plume during surgery.

Several wavelengths have been used in laser bronchoscopy. The CO_2 laser must be used through a rigid endoscope. This beam is not color-dependent, so there is uniform impact on all tissues. It is noted for its precise ablation with minimal adjacent tissue damage. This wavelength is not effective in treating highly vascular diseases. The Nd:YAG laser is used to treat diseases that require high penetration of laser energy such as tracheo–bronchial adenomas and obstructing carcinomas. This wavelength has excellent hemostatic abilities because of its 2 to 6 mm zone of thermal coagulation. The laser energy is delivered through a flexible fiber for use with a rigid or flexible endoscope. Safety issues in these cases revolve around eye safety for patient, placing a wet towel over the eyes, and the surgeon, wearing appropriate eyewear or using a special filter on the eyepiece of the endoscope to protect against backscatter. Teeth also need to be protected from injury and accidental beam impact. Additionally, fire is a concern during these cases. The flexible endoscopes are made of flammable material, and most cases are performed in an oxygen-rich environment that supports combustion [4].

The CO_2, contact Nd:YAG, or frequency doubled YAG lasers can be used to treat snoring. The laser-assisted uvula palatoplasty procedure alters the soft palate tissue to reduce the tissue's vibration. In nasal polypectomy, the KTP laser is used to debulk large multiple polyps, while the CO_2 laser vaporizes the polyps. Using the laser for removal of nasal polyps is less invasive than other techniques. In laser turbinectomy, the CO_2 and contact Nd:YAG laser vaporizes the superficial layer of mucosa without damaging the turbinate, while the KTP laser shrinks the turbinate without affecting the normal mucosa. Surgery in the middle ear has been enhanced, because laser energy can be delivered precisely to the structure and vaporizes tissue without vibratory movement. The CO_2, KTP, or Er:YAG lasers can be used for stapedotomy with insertion of a stapes prosthesis. A small opening into the footplate is accomplished by using low pulse energies. The laser energy is delivered to the tissue by a fiberoptic probe [4].

Gastroenterology

Today many institutions have designated suites where upper and lower gastrointestinal procedures are routinely performed. In esophageal obstructions from malignant tumors, the Nd:YAG and contact Nd:YAG lasers are being used to vaporize, excise or debulk the esophageal obstruction through an endoscope. This palliative procedure does not require an operating room environment and can be done locally or with intravenous sedation. Perforation is a complication of the procedure. In bleeding ulcers, the Nd:YAG laser is used to control bleeding in the gastric area because of its 2 to 6 mm depth of penetration.

Complications of this intervention are perforation and hemorrhage, which may require emergency surgery. Eye safety for the patient, surgeon, and team is critical when laser energy is being used through flexible endoscopes. The KTP, argon, and Nd:YAG lasers are used to treat colon or rectal polyps. Polyps or tumors less than 1 cm in diameter can be treated successfully with the argon or KTP lasers, while the Nd:YAG is needed for larger lesions. Obstructive colorectal tumors are treated palliatively like the obstructive esophageal tumors [5].

General

The CO_2 laser beam can be used to make the skin incision for a breast biopsy and mastectomy. During the breast biopsy, the lasers beam is used to raise a local flap. The defocused laser beam will coagulate small blood vessels. To excise the breast biopsy, the Nd:YAG laser can be used. In mastectomies, the CO_2 laser is being replaced by the contact Nd:YAG laser. Advantages of this laser include:

- The delivery system is less cumbersome that the articulating arm
- It restores tactile sensation to the surgeon
- It has less plume formation
- It has a control depth of penetration when cutting, coagulating, or vaporizing tissue

The CO_2 and contact Nd:YAG lasers are used in head and neck surgery such as parotidectomy, radical neck dissection, and thyroidectomy. These lasers provide hemostasis and sealing of the lymphatics. They reduce edema, decrease chance of spreading malignant cells to other parts of the body, and seal nerve endings. The contact Nd:YAG laser also has proven effective in procedures involving the pancreas, spleen, liver, and gall bladder. In laser hemorrhoidectomy, care must be taken with the presence of methane gas. The potential hazard of methane gas is the possibility of causing a lower bowel explosion or fire if the gas comes in contact with the lasers beam. A saline-soaked sponge can be packed into the lower rectal area to decrease the chance of the gas escaping during surgery. Any sponge that is packed into the rectum needs to be counted and removed at the end of the case. CO_2, argon, and KPT lasers use their energy as a cutting tool on third- and fourth-degree hemorrhoids. The CO_2 laser can be used to treat fissures, which usually are associated with hemorrhoids and fistulas. With a high anal fistula, the sphincter needs to be preserved, so a contact Nd:YAG laser also could be used [4].

Gynecology

Gynecologists were among the first specialists to realize the potentials of laser technology. Treatment for cervical intraepithelial neoplasia (CIN) is the conization and excision of the cervix. This can be accomplished by using a knife, cryosurgery, electrosurgery, or a laser. No matter which technique is used, the borders of the lesion need to be defined, and this is done by applying a 3%

solution of acetic acid to the cervix. Laser conization and vaporization are accomplished by coupling a CO_2 laser to a colposcope or operating microscope.

Contact Nd:YAG, argon, and frequency doubled YAG lasers also can be used for cervical excision and vaporization. Vulvar intraepithelial neoplasia (VIN) is treated with the CO_2 laser, if biopsies have confirmed that the disease is noninvasive. A solution of 3% acetic acid is applied to the lesions to delineate the margins. The laser is coupled to a colposcope or operating microscope, and the top layer of the dermis is vaporized superficially.

Condyloma acuminata, commonly referred to as genital or venereal warts, can be treated successfully with the CO_2, frequency doubled YAG, argon, and Nd:YAG lasers. The margins of the lesions are delineated with a 3% acetic acid. To enhance the visualization of the lesion, a colposcope, operating microscope, or loops can be used by the surgeon. Because the disease process is limited to the epidermal layer, deep vaporization of the dermis is not necessary. If intraepithelial neoplasia is suspected, however, deep tissue vaporization is recommended. The recurrence rate is reduced when treatment is with a laser, because the thermal energy helps destroys the surrounding viral contaminants. Because this disease is sexually transmitted, the sexual partner of the patient should be evaluated for condyloma acuminata. The human papilloma virus (HPV) can remain after treatment, so the virus still can be spread.

Many procedures that traditionally were open abdominal surgeries now are being accomplished as outpatient laparoscopic procedures. This surgical approach has led to fewer complications and more successful results, because the surgeon can cut and coagulate within the abdominal cavity without making a large incision. The addition of the laser to laparoscopic procedures allows for precise ablation/vaporization with minimal adjacent tissue damage, hemostasis, and less adhesion formation postoperatively. Originally, the CO_2 laser was coupled to the laparoscope, but this presented many problems with this delivery system. The laparoscope has evolved, accepting many different wavelengths and delivery systems. Endometriosis is caused by ectopic endometrial cells migrating out of the uterus to various sites throughout the pelvic and abdominal areas. Endometrial implants can be treated successfully during laparoscopy with less recurrence, because the laser beam can vaporize and excise most of the implants precisely. Because of the color selectivity of the laser beam, the argon, frequency doubled YAG, and Nd:YAG lasers are being used to treat these implants [4].

Various ovarian conditions, infertility, ectopic pregnancy, uterine fibroids, and adhesions can be treated with the CO_2, Nd:YAG, contact Nd:YAG, frequency double YAG, and argon lasers.

Endometrial ablation for menorrhagia or metrorrhagia can be accomplished by several modalities, including electrosurgical roller-ball, thermal balloon therapy, radio frequency, and the laser. If using a laser, the Nd:YAG is preferred because of the depth of penetration of its beam. The contact Nd:YAG, doubled YAG, and argon lasers also have been used, but their depth of beam penetration is not as good as the Nd:YAG.

Urology

CO_2, argon, Nd:YAG, contact YAG and frequency doubled YAG lasers are used to treat many urological conditions. Resection of bladder tumors through a scope can be accomplished with Nd:YAG or contact Nd:YAG lasers on an outpatient basis. During laser vaporization, the light energy of the beam seals the blood vessels and lymphatics. Because the laser does not create an electrical current through the irrigating fluid, the obturator nerve is not stimulated. The patient usually experiences less pain, does not need a catheter postoperatively, and recovers very quickly. Although recurrent bladder tumors are treated successfully with laser vaporization, research is being conducted on the use of the laser for invasive bladder tumors. Urethral strictures, a benign contraction of fibrous tissue secondary to trauma, inflammation or scarring, are being treated successfully with the Nd:YAG, contact Nd:YAG, frequency doubled YAG, Ho:YAG, and argon lasers.

An alternative therapy to extracorporeal shock wave lithotripsy (ESWL) and electrohydraulic lithotripsy (EHL) for treating ureteral calculi is laser lithotripsy. In this treatment, laser energy is delivered to the stone through a flexible or semirigid ureteroscope. The Ho:YAG and tunable pulse-dyed lasers are used, because their wavelength can disintegrate stones without damaging the adjacent tissue [5]. Normal saline solution is used as a continuous irrigation. Because of the smaller channels of the ureteroscopes, a pressure bag can be used to help with visualization and increase flow of the irrigation. After the stone is fragmented, it can be extracted from the ureter by various baskets or forceps designed for this purpose. These lasers also can be used to fragment stones in the bladder. Stone fragments should be sent for stone analysis.

Benign prostatic hypertrophy (BPH) is one of the most predominant reasons for surgery in older men. The traditional treatment for symptomatic BPH is an endoscopic transurethral resection of the prostate (TURP) using electrosurgery to resect only the periurethral adenomatous portion of the gland. This procedure requires a hospital admission of several days and has several complications, such as hematuria, prolonged catheterization, urinary tract infection, and recurrence of prostate enlargement.

TURP also can be accomplished using laser technology. The two most recent wavelengths to be used in the treatment of bladder outlet obstruction are the indigo and KTP lasers. A minimally invasive procedure, interstitial laser coagulation with the indigo laser is indicated for men older than 50 years with a median or lateral prostatic volume of 20 to 85 cc. This procedure can be performed safely in an office environment and designed for men who want to minimize their risk of incontinence or impotence [5]. The KTP laser is also effective in treating bladder outlet obstruction secondary to BPH. The KTP photoselective vaporization of the prostate (PVP) is performed as an outpatient procedure under general or spinal anesthesia. There is minimal to no blood loss, and no risk of transurethral resection syndrome, because there is essentially no fluid absorption during the case. The patient usually is discharged the same day without a catheter [13]. All patients, regardless of the prostate size, are candidates for the KTP photoselective vaporization of the prostate. Another alternate procedure for men who are sexually active with small-to-moderate obstructive prostate without a significant middle lobe is a transurethral incision of the prostate (TUIP). The prostate is incised at 5 and 7 o'clock using a KTP or contact Nd:YAG laser. This relieves the bladder neck obstruction with results similar to those done with a traditional TURP but with lower incidence of bladder neck contracture and retrograde ejaculation.

The CO_2, Nd:YAG, frequency doubled YAG, Ho:YAG, and argon lasers can be used to treat condylomata acuminata of the genitalia, including the meatal or periurethral areas. The treatment and outcomes are similar to the removal of these lesions from females. To decrease the chance of reinfection, a condom should be worn during sexual contact. Other procedures that use the Nd:YAG, or contact Nd:YAG are for partial or complete penile amputation for carcinoma, circumcision, vasectomy reversal, and partial nephrectomy.

LASER ECONOMICS AND LEGAL ISSUES

For lasers to remain a viable tool in the clinical setting, they must be cost-effective. The economics of the laser are dependent upon cost, charges, and reimbursement. All three areas must be assessed continually. Some hospitals are contracting a third party for laser cases. Renting precludes large investments of capital that would be needed for purchasing different wavelength lasers, and having their laser technician operate the laser frees a member of the surgical team. When using a third party vendor, the perioperative team is still responsible for the safe use of the laser in their environment, documentation on the perioperative record, and maintaining patient's confidentiality and privacy. In some instances, the use of a laser has been replaced by electrosurgery. Many surgeons feel it is a cheaper modality; specialized courses are not needed to learn its application, and no special credentials are needed. Physicians who use lasers need to be credentialed for each wavelength that they use. Health care providers who are involved with operating the laser must be qualified and have documentation on file. Yearly refresher courses should be given to staff members who run the laser to maintain their competency.

SUMMARY

Lasers have made a significant impact on surgery since their introduction into medicine. All specialties have benefited from this technology. Surgeries that once were not possible to perform now can be done safely with lasers. The knowledge base and responsibilities for the safe use of lasers continue to grow as new wavelengths are developed and perfected for clinical use. Their possibilities are limitless. Through all this technology, the perioperative nurse will continue to be the patient's advocate by providing a safe environment during surgery.

References

[1] MacKety CJ. Perioperative laser nursing. A practical guide. Cincinnati (OH): Lasers of America; 1989.

[2] Ball KA. Lasers in the OR. Thorofare (NJ): Slack Inc; 1988.

[3] Ball KA. Lasers. The perioperative challenge. St. Louis (MO): Mosby; 1990.

[4] Ball KA. Lasers. The perioperative challenge. 2nd edition. St. Louis (MO): Mosby; 1995.

[5] Rothrock JC, editor. Alexander's care of the patient in surgery. 12th edition. St. Louis (MO): Mosby; 2003.

[6] Dorsey JH. Education and credentialing of the gynecology laser surgeon. Obstet Gynecol Clin North Am 1991;18:661–5.

[7] Champion J. Laser safety management. Br J Perioper Nurs 2000;10:428–32.

[8] Youker SR, Ammirati CT. Practical aspects of laser safety. Journal of Facial Plastic Surgery 2001;17:155–63.

[9] Andersen K. Safe use of lasers in the operating room—what perioperative nurses should know. AORN J 2004;79:171–88.

[10] Sosis MB. Evaluation of a new laser-resistant operating room drape, eye shield, and anesthesia circuit protector. J Clin Laser Med Surg 1993;11:255–7.

[11] Fortunato N. Berry & Kohn's operating room technique. 9th edition. St. Louis (MO): Mobsy; 2000.

[12] Houck PM, Cooke TR, Emanuel C. Laser applications in orthopedics. Semin Perioper Nurs 1993;2:82–9.

[13] Muller N, Muller EJ. KTP photoselective laser vaporization of the prostate: indications, procedure, and nursing implications. Urol Nurs 2004;24:373–8.

Nurs Clin N Am 41 (2006) 219–229

NURSING CLINICS
OF NORTH AMERICA

Laparoscopy: Risks, Benefits and Complications

Diana L. Wadlund, RN, CRNFA, CRNP

Surgical Specialists, 1351 Julieanna Drive, West Chester, PA 19380, USA

L aparoscopic surgery is a minimally invasive alternative to traditional laparotomy. It is used as a diagnostic measure and for performing minor and major operative surgical procedures. Many procedures that traditionally were performed using open laparotomy now are being accomplished laparoscopically. There are numerous benefits to laparoscopy, including smaller incisions, decreased hospital stay, and decreased recovery time. Laparoscopy also allows the surgeon better visualization and magnification of anatomy and pathology [1].

Laparoscopy does have certain risks and complications, most of which are associated with entry into the abdominal cavity. These complications can have a major impact on the patient's outcome [2].

This article discusses the benefits and risks of laparoscopy. Also discussed are complications of laparoscopy and methods to avoid or treat these adversities.

PATIENT SELECTION

Indications for laparoscopic surgery are the same as for the equivalent open procedure. The goal of laparoscopy is to perform the surgical procedure in a similar manner as the standard technique without opening the peritoneal cavity [1].

There are two absolute contraindications to laparoscopy: the patient's inability to tolerate general anesthesia, and the surgeon's inexperience and lack of skill with the specific procedure or technique [3].

Laparoscopy allows for decreased morbidity, decreased hospital stay, and improved cosmetic results. Conversion from laparoscopy to laparotomy is a double-edged sword. The patient has the expense of the laparoscopic procedure and a larger incision with resultant increased pain and recovery time. Although it is impossible to consistently predict the likelihood of conversion from laparoscopy to an open procedure, a few guidelines exist [3].

Patients who have had prior abdominal surgery have an increased likelihood of abdominal adhesion formation. Tissue planes may be distorted or

E-mail address: dlw522@aol.com

0029-6465/06/$ – see front matter
doi:10.1016/j.cnur.2006.01.003

impossible to identify. The experienced surgeon will have gained skill in lysis of adhesions and identifying difficult tissue planes through the laparoscope. He also will realize his surgical limitations and will open in a timely and appropriate manner when it is necessary [1].

OBESE PATIENTS

Obese patients provide many challenges to the operative surgeon, and the use of laparoscopy is no exception. Obesity was once an absolute contraindication for laparoscopy. Trocar and instrument depth were often too shallow to reach the operative site.

Advances in instrumentation have provided the surgeon with the means to use laparoscopic techniques on the obese patient. In reality, laparoscopy provides numerous benefits for the obese patient, including:

- Access to the surgical site is often easier, and visualization of the anatomy vastly improved with the use of the laparoscope.
- Large incisions required for certain open surgical procedures are often even larger in the obese patient to allow for adequate visualization.
- Recovery time is reduced greatly with minimally invasive surgery, decreasing the risk for potentially devastating complications [2].

Other relative contraindications include severe portal hypertension, coagulopathy, and diffuse carcinomatosis in the abdomen [2].

Patients should be evaluated medically before laparoscopy and laparotomy, with specific attention focused on cardiac and pulmonary status. If a patient is medically unfit to undergo laparotomy, he or she should not undergo elective laparoscopy.

PREGNANT PATIENTS

Laparoscopy on the pregnant patient may be wrought with potential peril. There are certainly risks associated with anesthesia, radiologic patient evaluation, and laparoscopy, but studies have shown that most of the morbidity and mortality associated with surgical problems in the obstetric patient and in the fetus is secondary to the underlying disease process [4]. Certain things, however, should be considered, such as:

- Length of gestation
- Open versus blind laparoscopic technique to avoid injury to the gravid uterus
- The physiologic effects of the CO_2 on the fetus
- Alternations in technique because of the presence of the enlarged uterus [4]

The most common indications for laparoscopic surgery in the pregnant patient are appendicitis, cholelithiasis, and ectopic pregnancy. Technically, laparoscopy should occur during the second trimester, ideally before 23 weeks, to minimize risk of preterm labor and to have adequate intra-abdominal working room. This allows ease in placing the insufflation needle or Hasson trocar and visualization of the appendix or gallbladder. The open laparoscopic technique to establish pneumoperitoneum is the safest method to avoid injury to intra-abdominal organs. After the second trimester, an open laparotomy would be a safer technique [4].

During the surgical procedure certain guidelines should be followed. The mother's acid base balance and end-tidal CO_2 should be monitored. The patient should be rolled 30° to the left side to avoid compression of the inferior vena cava (IVC). Intra-abdominal pressure should be limited to between 8 and 12 mm Hg. The fetal heart rate should be monitored during anesthesia induction and periodically throughout the procedure [1,4].

SURGICAL PROCEDURE

The first step in the laparoscopy is establishment of pneumoperitoneum. There are two techniques used to establish pneumoperitoneum: the closed technique and the open technique.

Closed Technique

The closed technique involves use of an insufflation needle. János Veres invented an insufflation needle, which is an automatic, spring-loaded, dual needle. The blunt inner portion of the Veress needle is pushed back by the resistance of the skin, allowing the sharp outer portion to easily puncture the skin. Once through the skin, resistance from skin and soft tissue is lost, and the blunt inner portion springs forward to prevent injury to internal organs [5,6].

The technique for inserting the Veress needle involves placing the patient in Trendelenburg (head down) position to displace the small bowel from the pelvis, elevating the anterior abdominal wall, and inserting the needle at a 45° angle pointed inferiorly [6].

After the abdomen is insufflated with CO_2 to an intra-abdominal pressure of 12 to 18 mm/Hg, the Veress needle is removed, the incision enlarged, and a 10 mm Trocar inserted into the abdomen.

Although precautions are taken to avoid injury to the intra-abdominal organs, the insufflation needle approach to establishing pneumoperitoneum is still a blind technique. Complications can occur because of lack of visualization of intra-abdominal organs [7,8]. Also, if the patient has any intra-abdominal adhesions to the anterior abdominal wall, a fact that cannot predicted with even the slightest degree of certainty, there is a greater risk for complications.

Open Technique

The open laparoscopic technique involves placement of a Hasson trocar. The Hasson trocar is a blunt tip trocar designed to be inserted using the open laparoscopic technique.

This technique involves making a small incision near the patient's umbilicus and placing two stitches into the patient's external oblique fascia. The two stitches then are lifted and an incision made between them through the fascia and into the peritoneum under direct visualization. The Hasson Trocar then is inserted into the opening in the abdominal wall and adhered securely to the abdominal wall using the two fascial stitches. Although the open technique for establishing pneumoperitoneum is technically safer than the closed technique, inadvertent injury to the abdominal contents can still occur.

Insufflation of the peritoneal cavity follows placement of the Veress needle or the Hasson trocar. Insufflation is necessary, because the abdomen is filled with organs that take up all the available space. Without insufflation, there is no room to visualize anatomy or perform a surgical intervention.

After pneumoperitoneum has been established, other trocars are placed into the abdomen under direct visualization. Direct visualization involves using a laparoscope to watch a trocar being inserted through the abdominal wall. This decreases the risk of visceral injury.

PNEUMOPERITONEUM

Pneumoperitoneum is achieved by infusing CO_2 into the peritoneal cavity. CO_2 is the agent of choice for establishing pneumoperitoneum for gynecologic and general surgical procedures. CO_2 is more soluble in blood than air, oxygen, or N_2O. CO_2 is also accessible and inexpensive; it suppresses combustion and is eliminated rapidly, increasing its margin of safety [9].

A few disadvantages of CO_2 include increased peritoneal irritation with increased postoperative discomfort and an increased risk for cardiac arrhythmia. CO_2 is tolerated poorly by patients with impaired pulmonary function [9].

In its infancy 20 to 30 years ago, laparoscopy was performed on young healthy individuals. The intra-abdominal pressure (IAP) could be as high as 40 mm Hg with no adverse effects on the patient. Currently, the intra-abdominal pressure is kept at 12 to 18 mm/Hg, which is a much safer level for the older, more medically and physiologically debilitated patients treated today [3].

Pneumoperitoneum causes certain physiologic changes. These changes are based on such things as IAP, amount of CO_2 absorbed, circulatory volume of the patient, ventilatory technique used, underlying pathology, and type of anesthesia [3]. Table 1 discusses the effects of pneumoperitoneum on several body systems [1].

PULMONARY EFFECTS

Increased intra-abdominal volume and pressure impede diaphragmatic excursion. Patient positioning does not alter the effects of insufflation on pulmonary function. Table 1 outlines the physiologic effects of pneumoperitoneum on the pulmonary system.

Because the minimally invasive nature of laparoscopic surgery, the patient has less pain and subsequently fewer pulmonary issues postoperatively when compared with open procedures [1].

CIRCULATORY EFFECTS

Healthy individuals are under no threat from the cardiovascular effects of peritoneal insufflation. Patients with impaired compensatory mechanisms, however, do not tolerate the effects of laparoscopy [1].

Most patients can have a safe laparoscopic experience with careful monitoring, proper fluid balance, and prompt attention to problems that arise. Patients with severely impaired cardiac function are served better with an open procedure [1].

Physiologic effects of pneumoperitoneum on the circulatory system are outlined in Table 1. Physiologic change is affected by patient positioning. For example, the Trendelenburg position increases intra-thoracic pressure, central venous pressure, capillary wedge pressure, and mean arterial pressure, thus increasing cardiac work load. Reverse Trendelenburg leads to decreased cardiac output by decreasing preload, possibly causing hypotension [1].

Table 1
Physiologic effects of pneumoperitoneum and potential clinical outcomes

Organ system	Physiologic effects	Potential outcomes
Pulmonary	↑ Peak airway pressures	Barotrauma/pneumothorax
	↓ Pulmonary compliance and vital capacity	↑ Pco_2 and/or ↓ Po_2
	Superior displacement of the diaphragm	↑ Pco_2 and/or ↓ Po_2
	↑ End-tidal CO_2	Acidosis
Circulatory	Direct effects—increased CVP, CWP, SVR, MAP	↑ Cardiac work; effects on cardiac output dependent on volume status
	Indirect effects of CO_2—arteriolar dilation and myocardial depression	↓ Blood pressure
	Indirect effects on the sympathetic system, renin-angiotensin system, and vasopressin	↑ Blood pressure and cardiac output
		↓ Urine output
Renal	↓ Renal blood flow	↓ Urine output
Coagulation	Lower extremity venous stasis	DVT and PE
Immunity and inflammation	Preserved systemic immunity	Greater resistance to infection and tumor seeding
	Impaired local immunity	↓ Resistance to infection or tumor seeding
Central nervous system	↑ ICP	↓ Central perfusion pressure
Intestinal	Attenuated sympathetic response	Less ileus

Abbreviations: CVP, central venous pressure; CWP, capillary wedge pressure; DVT, deep venous pressure; ICP, intracranial pressure; MAP, mean arterial pressure; PE, pulmonary embolus; SVR, systemic vascular resistance.

From Philips PA, Amaral JF. Abdominal access complications in laparoscopic surgery. J Am Coll Surg 2001;192(4):525–36; with permission.

RENAL EFFECTS

Urine output is lower with pneumoperitoneum than with open laparotomy. Oliguria is common during long laparoscopic procedures. Increased intra-abdominal pressure leads to decreased renal blood flow [1].

COMPLICATIONS OF PNEUMOPERITONEUM

Cardiovascular

Hypercarbia and acidosis result from CO_2 absorption and can lead to myocardial irritability. Cardiac dysrhythmia, specifically ventricular ectopy, can occur [9].

Extraperitoneal Insufflation

Extraperitoneal insufficiency can occur because of an improperly placed Veress needle, resulting in subcutaneous emphysema. CO_2 emphysema resolves promptly after insufflation ceases [9]. Inadvertent insufflation of intra-abdominal structures such as omentum or mesentery can obscure the visibility of intra-abdominal structures, increasing the risk of injury to them [3].

Pneumothorax/Pneumomediastinum/Pneumopericardium

During the creation of pneumoperitoneum, the movement of gas can produce pneumomediastinum, unilateral pneumothorax, bilateral pneumothorax, and pneumopericardium. These maladies occur for several reasons. Embryonic remnants that allow potential channels of communication between the abdomen and the chest open because of increased intra-abdominal pressure. Defects in the diaphragm and weak points in the aorta and esophageal hiatus may allow passage of gas into the thorax. Pleural tears that can occur because of laparoscopic surgical technique at the level of the GE (gastro–esophageal) junction can result in pneumothorax. Opening of peritoneopleural ducts can result mainly in right-sided pneumothorax. Pneumothorax during fundoplication is noted more frequently on the left side [9].

Potentially serious complications associated with pneumoperitoneum may lead to respiratory and hemodynamic disturbances. Capnothorax (CO_2 pneumothorax) decreases thoraco–pulmonary compliance, increases airway pressures, and increases PaO_2 and $PETCO_2$ [9].

CO_2 absorption is greater from the pleural cavity than from the peritoneal cavity. Tension pneumothorax with cardio–respiratory compromise can occur [9]. When CO_2 pneumothorax occurs during laparoscopy, several guidelines are followed:

- Stop N_2O administration.
- Correct hypoxemia, adjust ventilator.
- Apply PEEP (positive end-expiratory pressure).
- Decrease intra-abdominal pressure.
- Pneumothorax usually resolves promptly after exsufflation; thoracocentesis should be avoided.
- In the case of a preexisting bullae rupturing, PEEP and thoracocentesis should be applied [9].

GAS EMBOLISM

Gas embolism is a rare but very dangerous complication of laparoscopy. Gas embolism can be caused by needle or trocar placement into a vessel or insufflation into an abdominal organ [9].

Physiologically, rapid insufflation of gas under high pressure causes a gas obstruction of the vena cava or atrium. Decreased cardiac output, circulatory collapse, and obstruction to venous return can occur. In patients who have patent foramen ovale, 20% to 30% of the population, right ventricular hypertension can open the foramen, allowing gas embolism of the cerebral and coronary beds [9].

Diagnosis is obtained by detecting gas embolism on the right side of the heart or in recognizing physiologic changes. In events occurring with 0.5 mL/kg or air or less, changes will be noted in Doppler sounds and increased mean pulmonary arterial pressure. When embolism increases in size to 2 mL/kg of air, signs and symptoms include:

- Tachycardia
- Hypotension
- Increased central venous pressure
- Mill wheel cardiac murmur,
- Cyanosis
- Flash pulmonary edema
- Cardiac arrhythmia and
- EKG changes consistent with right heart strain [9]

Treatment includes:

- Immediate cessation of insufflation and release of pneumothorax
- Place patient in steep Trendelenburg on left side to prevent gas from entering the pulmonary outflow tract.
- Discontinue N_2O and ventilate with 100% oxygen. The high solubility of CO_2 in blood results in rapid absorption of CO_2 from the blood, allowing for rapid reversal of signs and symptoms.
- Aspiration of gas with a central venous catheter
- External cardiac massage to fragment large bubbles [9]

TECHNICAL COMPLICATIONS

Laparoscopic complications occur at a rate of approximately 4 to 6 complications per 1000 patients, with a mortality rate of approximately 3 deaths per 100,000 patients. The more complex laparoscopic procedures result in a higher risk for complications. Box 1 lists some complications of laparoscopy [1].

Vascular Injuries

Although vascular complications are rare, with an incidence of 0.02% to 0.03%, there is a significant mortality rate of 15% [1]. Injuries to intra-abdominal vascular structures with the insufflation needle or trocar placement are the

Box 1: General complications of laparoscopy

Injury to adjacent organs

Bleeding from solid organs (liver and spleen)

Vascular injuries

Puncture/perforation/cauterization of the bowel

Transection/perforation of bile ducts

Perforation of the bladder

Puncture/perforation of the uterus

Complications of abdominal access

- Port site hernia
- Wound infection
- *Also see* Injury to adjacent organs

Complications of specimen removal

Port site recurrence of cancer

Splenosis

Endometriosis

Complications of pneumoperitoneum

- Pneumothorax
- Pneumomediastinum
- Gas embolus
- Subcutaneous emphysema

From Philips PA, Amaral JF. Abdominal access complications in laparoscopic surgery. J Am Coll Surg 2001;192(4):525–36; with permission.

most threatening laparoscopic complication [2,7]. Vascular injuries can be prevented by:

- Evaluation of anterior abdominal wall
- Proper patient positioning—Trendelenburg—when placing the insufflation needle or a trocar
- Insertion of insufflation needle or a trocar at the correct angle, 45° angle directed caudally
- Using the open laparoscopic technique with use of the Hasson trocar [1]

Large vessel injuries occur during laparoscopic access. The right common iliac artery is the most commonly injured blood vessel because of its location directly below the umbilicus. Box 2 discusses factors responsible for large vessel injury during laparoscopic access [1].

Lateral to the abdominal wall midline are blood vessels: superior epigastrics, inferior epigastrics, and superior circumflex iliac vessels. These vascular structures can be injured when placing lateral trocars. In most patients,

---

Box 2: Factors responsible for large-vessel injury during laparoscopic access

Inexperienced or unskilled surgeon

Failure to sharpen the trocar

Failure to place the patient in Trendelenburg position

Failure to elevate or stabilize the abdominal wall

Perpendicular insertion of the needle or trocar

Lateral deviation of the needle or trocar

Inadequate pneumoperitoneum

Forceful thrust

Failure to note anatomic landmarks

Inadequate incision size

From Philips PA, Amaral JF. Abdominal access complications in laparoscopic surgery. J Am Coll Surg 2001;192(4):525–36; with permission.

---

transillumination of the anterior abdominal wall will allow for visualization of these structures. Sometimes abdominal wall thickness disallows visibility of theses structures. In that case, it is advised to place the lateral trocars approximately 8 cm from the midline and at least 5 cm from the symphysis pubis to avoid injury to the abdominal wall blood vessels [2].

Bowel Injuries

Potentially catastrophic injury can occur to the gastrointestinal tract during trocar placement. One contributing factor to potential bowel injury is prior abdominal surgery. It is estimated that approximately 25% of patients with midline abdominal incisions from prior surgery have periumbilical adhesions [1].

One study reveals that the incidence of bowel injury during gynecologic laparoscopy ranged from 0.08% to 0.33%. As many as 15% of these injuries were not discovered until several days postoperatively, with one out of five resulting in death [8]. In yet another study by Chandler and colleagues, reviewing general and gynecologic procedures, 76% of all injuries incurred during the establishment of the primary port were bowel and retroperitoneal vascular in nature. Nearly 50% of the injuries to the small and large intestine went unrecognized for at least 24 hours [7].

In the patient who has midline abdominal scars, an alternate site for entry into the abdomen should be considered. The left upper quadrant rarely has adhesions and would provide an excellent view of the periumbilical region to evaluate for bowel adhesions [1].

Although it seems logical that the use of the open laparoscopic technique would be safer, statistically there is no difference between use of the insufflation needle and the Hasson trocar [10].

Bowel burns can occur during laparoscopy, resulting in the need for open laparotomy and possible colostomy. The use of the new harmonic scalpel, bipolar cauterization techniques, and methods that use surgical clips or staples helps to minimize this risk [11].

Delayed diagnosis of these injuries is an independent predictor of mortality [8]. When major abdominal procedures are being performed, patients should be instructed to do a preoperative antibiotic bowel preparation to reduce the incidence of peritonitis caused by inadvertent bowel injury [12,13].

Urologic Injuries

Injuries to the ureter have occurred as a consequence of thermal injury, ligation, or laceration caused by inadequate exposure or poor dissection. Bladder injury can occur with trocar placement. Placement of a Foley catheter can help decrease the size of the bladder, thus decreasing the risk of perforation [14].

Studies have demonstrated that the risk of injury correlates positively with the degree of complexity of the surgical procedure. Proper identification of anatomic structures and surgical planes is mandatory to avoid injury [2].

Small injuries to the bladder such as a Veress needle stick can be managed with bladder decompression. Larger injuries induced by a trocar stick or dissection require open laparotomy with repair of the injury [8,11].

WOUND COMPLICATIONS
Hernia

Hernias occur in 0.1% to 0.3% of patients. Larger trocars pose a greater the risk for herniation. When using a 10 mm or larger trocar, the patient's fascia should be sutured closed to avoid possible herniation [3].

Wound Infection

It is uncommon for a wound infection to occur, and risk depends largely on the type of surgical procedure performed. Diagnostic laparoscopy has an extremely low wound infection rate approximately 0.1%. Wound infections following laparoscopic cholecystectomy, for example, can be as high as 1%, however [3]. Use of the bag or other device to remove the specimen may decrease the incidence of infection [3].

SUMMARY

When laparoscopic surgery was in its infancy, many said that it was a temporary phenomenon, a passing phase on the surgical timeline. Tincture of time has proven the efficacy of laparoscopic surgery, and advances in laparoscopic surgery have altered the way surgery is viewed and performed. Attention to the detail of proper patient selection, use of appropriate surgical technique, and prompt management of surgical complications can ensure that the minimally invasive nature of laparoscopic surgery remains the outcome for most if not all laparoscopic patients. Perioperative nursing care plans must be in place to address possible complications such uncontrollable intraoperative bleeding or adverse occurrences such as pneumothorax [15].

References

[1] Chang C, Rege RV. Minimally invasive surgery. In: Townsend CM, et al, editors. Sabiston textbook of surgery. 17th edition. Philadelphia: WB Saunders; 2004.

[2] Levie MD. Laparoscopic complications and their prevention. Available at: http://www.medscape.com. Accessed February 15, 2006.

[3] Modlin IM, Begos DG, Ballantyne GH. What's new in laparoscopic surgery. In: Spiro HM, editor. Clinical Gastroenterology, 1994;(Suppl 1):1–20

[4] Melnick DM, Wahl WL, Dalton VK. Management of general surgical problems in the pregnant patient. Am J Surg 2004;187(2).

[5] Szabo I, Laszio A. Veress needle: in memoriam of the 100th birthday anniversary of Dr. János Veres, the inventor. Am J Obstet Gynecol 2004;191(1):352–3.

[6] Vilos GA, Vilos AG. Safe laparoscopic entry guided by Veres needle CO_2 insufflation pressure. J Minim Invasive Gynecol 2003;10(3):415–20.

[7] Chandler JG, Corson SL, Way LW. Three spectra of laparoscopic entry access injuries. J Am Coll Surg 2001;192(4):478–90.

[8] Brosens I, Gordon A, Campo R, et al. Bowel injury in gynecologic laparoscopy. J Minim Invasive Gynecol 2003;10(1):9–13.

[9] Joris JL. Anesthesia for laparoscopic surgery. In Miller RD: Miller's Anesthesia, ed. 6, Philadelphia, 2005: 2285–2299, Elsevier.

[10] Neudecker J, et al. The European Association for Endoscopic Surgery: Clinical practice guideline on pneumoperitoneum for laparoscopic surgery. Surg Endosc 2002;16(7): 1121–43.

[11] Hurd WW, Duke JM, Harris CM. Gynecologic laparoscopy. Available at: www.emedicine.com/med/topic3299.htm. Accessed February 15, 2006.

[12] Georgia Reproductive Specialists. Laparoscopy. Available at: www.ivf.com/laprscpy.html. Accessed February 15, 2006.

[13] Gruendemann BJ, Mangum SS. Infection prevention in surgical settings. Philadelphia: WB Saunders; 2001.

[14] Armenakas NA, Pareek G, Fracchia JA. Iatrogenic bladder perforations: long-term follow-up of 65 patients. J Am Coll Surg 2004;198(1):78–82.

[15] Rothrock JC. Alexander's care of the patient in surgery. 12th edition. St. Louis (MO): Mosby; 2003.

Nurs Clin N Am 41 (2006) 231–248

NURSING CLINICS
OF NORTH AMERICA

How Religion, Language and Ethnicity Impact Perioperative Nursing Care

Donna M. DeFazio Quinn, BSN, MBA, RN, CPAN, CAPA*

Orthopaedic Surgery Center, 264 Pleasant Street, Concord, NH 03301, USA

Religion, language, and ethnicity play important roles in the perioperative arena. Each nurse carries his or her own individualized sociocultural background and beliefs to the organization. Awareness of own beliefs, as well as those of the patients served, is essential in the perioperative area. With the United States becoming a melting pot of cultural diversity, perioperative nurses must possess the skills and knowledge necessary to deal with the conglomeration of vast differences in patient population [1].

RELIGION

Spiritual and religious beliefs play an important role in the perioperative arena [2]. Each patient brings an individualized preference to meet his or her spiritual or religious beliefs. The perioperative nurse must use astute observation and perception to recognize those patients who would benefit from spiritual or religious intervention during the perioperative period. Some patients have rules and beliefs concerning how health care is received. For example, some patients believe in burning candles, blessing the throat to prevent illnesses, baptism to cleanse of evil, and circumcision as a covenant to be loyal to God.

For some religious sects, the religious beliefs of the patient are tied closely to the decision to undergo surgery [3]. The religious beliefs of the patient may be tied closely to how the patient views illness, impending surgery, and treatment. Some religious groups rely on the clergy to assist and guide them and their families in the decision-making process. Others may use the services of a healer from their community. Prayer and ritualistic ceremonies such as the laying on of hands may be used to assist in the healing process.

In nonemergent situations, the perioperative nurse has the ability to discuss with and assist the patient in using religious and spiritual practices before surgery. Some of the practices that may be employed are outlined in Table 1.

*10 Foster Hill Road, Henniker, NH 03242, USA. *E-mail address:* dquinn@crhc.org

0029-6465/06/$ – see front matter
doi:10.1016/j.cnur.2006.01.002 nursing.theclinics.com

Table 1
Implication of ethnicity and religion on nursing interventions

Ethnicity/religion	Denominations/values	Nursing interventions
African American	• Strong religious orientation • Generally of Protestant faith • Frequently use prayer as a means to treat illness	• Religion may be an escape from the harsh realities of life. • A minister may assist in bridging the gap between the patient and the health care providers.
American Eskimo	• Inuit Indian • Christian • Language was Inuktituk, written in symbols; now speak several languages	• View death as a normal part of life • High alcohol consumption • High unemployment • May believe in spirits
Amish	• Considered a conservative Christian faith with Anabaptist tradition (rebaptism) • Started as reform group of Mennonite movement	• Folk medical practices and opposition to healthcare dominant in some families • Modern western medical interventions directly conflict with beliefs, complicating care
Appalachian	• Episcopalian or some other form of organized denomination • Very religious in that they value religion	• Family values are very important; it is essential to obtain family opinions and attitudes with regard to care and interventions in order to gain acceptance. • Entire family may gather to be with the patient. • Include family members in patient teaching. • Religious beliefs may influence the patients decision to seek medical care and treatment.
Chinese American	• Taoism, Buddhism, Islam, and Christianity	• Family oriented; the patient may put family before personal concerns • Family is based on hierarchical structure. • Incorporate family members into the plan of care. • Language barriers may prevent patient from following specified treatment regimens. • May incorporate herbal treatments and over-the-counter medications with prescribed medications • May incorporate traditional practices such as acupuncture and herbal treatments to restore balance to the body (yin and yang) • Believe certain foods have yin and yang properties

Table 1 (continued)		
Ethnicity/religion	Denominations/values	Nursing interventions
East Indian American	• Hindu religion	• Teachings emphasize truthfulness, self-control and respect for others • Commonly engage in meditation, singing, yoga, and daily prayer • Engage in daily prayer to the gods, usually early morning and early evening • Engage in fasting on certain days of the week • Father is regarded as head of family and is the primary spokesperson. • Wife will not participate in healthcare teachings; information is directed to the husband.
French Canadian	• Wide variety of religions—Catholic, Protestant, Judaism, Buddhist, Islam, Hindu, and Seventh-Day Adventist	• Declining national health budget (Canadian) increases reliance on community services. • Diverse ethnic and cultural groups in large cities require the nurse to be aware of various cultural practices.
Haitian American	• Voodoo, Christianity	• Rely on readers who predict the future through reading cards or hands and cure through the voodoo spirit • View illness as a hex or evil curse placed on them
Irish American	• Predominantly Catholic	• Family and family structure are very important. • Involve family in care and treatment plan. • Tend to wait until the last possible moment to seek medical assistance • Inherent not to adhere to schedules—important to emphasize need to adhere to schedules in regards to treatments and medication administration
Japanese American	• Tend to adopt the religion predominant in their area • Cultural values are derived from Zen Buddhism, Confucianism, and Shintoism	• Family plays a significant role. • May provide a bedside vigil to the hospitalized patient • Men may expect their wives or daughters to serve in the caretaker role so as to not bother the nurse.

Table 1
(continued)

Ethnicity/religion	Denominations/values	Nursing interventions
		• Confidentiality and respect are highly important; patient information should not be shared with extended family members, even those close to the patient.
Jehovah's Witness	• Considered a withdrawal group • Believe that personal experience and commitment are more important than the family	• Opposed to homologous blood transfusion, may agree to certain types of autologous transfusions • May allow certain blood volume expanders • Patients may refuse surgical and medical interventions for self and family members • In the United States, the general consensus is that an adult patient has the right to refuse treatment, but treatment cannot be withheld from a minor.
Jewish American	• Judaism	• Family involvement very important • Generally seek the opinion or two, three or four physicians before deciding on treatment • Want to know everything involved in their treatment • Will seek complete information regarding drug therapy (ie, purpose, edverse effects) • Consider it important to express their feelings; complaining is generally an accepted and expected practice • Patient may be very verbal during illness) (ie, crying and moaning). • Maintaining a kosher diet may present a challenge. • Identity has changed throughout generations, most do not observe traditional Sabbath.
Korean American	• Combination of Shamanism, Taoism, Buddhism, Confucianism and Christianity • Korean Americans harmonize both and practice in a Christian manner	• Very family oriented • Include family members in the plan of care. • Awareness that patients may utilize modern medical treatments in conjunction with traditional herbal remedies

Table 1
(continued)

Ethnicity/religion	Denominations/values	Nursing interventions
Latter Day Saints (LDS)	• Mormon • Same teachings and basic organization as established in the New Testament by Christ • Observe full religious lifestyle of attendance, devotion, service, learning • Believe physical body is gift from God • Believe obedience to health laws enhances physical, mental, and spiritual well-being • God mandates striving to achieve and maintain optimum health.	• Avoid habit-forming agents such as alcohol, tobacco, coffee, tea • Use meat sparingly; emphasis on fruits, vegetables, herbs, grains, and fish • Allowance for two priests to bless patient by laying on of hands and anoint patient with consecrated olive oil preoperatively • Decision regarding receiving or donating blood is individual. • Organ donation and transplantation are individual decisions. • Sabbath is day of rest and worship. • May reject pain medication
Mennonite	• Anabaptist Christian faith • Bible considered scared text, especially the New Testament • The Third Way family of European Free Church	• May consider the Last Supper as ordinance for foot washing • Have personal relationship with God • Pastoral community
Mexican Americans	• Predominantly Roman Catholic	• Spiritual healing and prayer very common • May have a Mexican folk healer visit (curandero) • Patient and family will have more respect for caregivers who accept the spiritual beliefs and understand the role of the curandero. • Curandero relieves people of their sins thereby allowing healing. • Patients may wear amulets to protect against evil and evil spirits.
Muslim [28]	• Islam • Qur'an (holy book) prohibits eating pork, meat of dead animals, blood, and intoxicants. • Muslim/Kosher meals • Fast 1 month a year • Autopsy not permitted	• Use prayer and patience to deal with illness • Illness is atonement for sins. • Consider death part of journey toward the Lord; follow Islamic guidelines for funeral preparation • May request their Imam to visit them • Do not insist on autopsy or organ donation • Provide same-sex health care person.

Table 1
(continued)

Ethnicity/religion	Denominations/values	Nursing interventions
Native American Indian	• Guided by sacred myths and legends • Approximately 50 tribes throughout the United States such as Navajo, Hopi, Sioux (Dakota), Apache, Arapaho, Cree, Crow, Osage, and Comanche	• Extended family may be present to care for the patient. • Nurse needs to understand the significance of the clan system among specific tribe. • Incorporate many cultural practices to bring harmony • Nurse needs to determine which cultural acts do not interfere with Western medicine and incorporate these into the plan of care.
Phillipino American	• Predominantly Roman Catholic	• May believe that disease and illness are the will of God • Continue to hope and pray for a cure even in dire situations • Patients generally do not complain and suffer in silence. • Family is very important, many may live together. • Many family members may hover over the patient.
Russian American	• Mainly Eastern Orthodox	• Requires fast days and abstinence from meat on Wednesday and Friday • During Lent, all animal products are forbidden (includes dairy). • Need to incorporate the entire family into the plan of care. • Elderly and immigrants may practice homeopathic or folk medicine. • Important to seek advice and opinion from the father before presenting plan of care to the rest of the family • Rarely submit to donation of organs because to religious beliefs • Do not inform patient of impending death; inform the head of the family.
Seventh-Day Adventist	• Considered a withdrawal group • Believe that personal experience and commitment are more important than the family	• Requires the nurse to have knowledge of the religious doctrines of the church • Believe that the body should be kept healthy • May refuse surgery and medical interventions on a Friday evening or Saturday because direct conflict with religious doctrines • Dietary restrictions include items such as seafood with shells, certain fish (eg, scavenger fish), meat, caffeine, alcohol, drugs, and tobacco

	Table 1 (continued)	
Ethnicity/religion	Denominations/values	Nursing interventions

Society of Friends	• Quaker: four movements
	  ○ Friends General Conference
	  ○ Orthodox Friends United Meeting
	  ○ Evangelical Friends International
	  ○ Conservative Meeting
	• Four styles of worship
	• Roots in radical Puritanism
	• Opposed to racism, sexism, religious intolerance
	• Believe Bible is a guide and not for literal interpretation
		• Ritualistic
		• Adapt well to outside beliefs without altering their own
		• May have pastoral leadership depending on particular sect
		• Not dependent on priests or ministers for spiritual guidance
		• Individual relationship with God

Vietnamese American	• Mainly a combination of the three traditional religions of Vietnam: Buddhism, Confucianism, and Taoism	• When death is imminent, the parents or head of family are informed first. • A priest or monk may be asked to visit. • Family may cry loudly while others pray. • Include family in the plan of care • Rarely submit to organ donation due to religious beliefs • In a hospital situation, a visit by the clergy is viewed as facing a grave situation.

Adapted from Giger JN, Davihizar RE. Transcultural nursing: assessment and intervention. 4th edition. St. Louis (MO): Elsevier; 2004.

It is important for the nurse to recognize when a patient is feeling spiritual distress. The patient may verbalize statement such as "Why did God do this to me?" It is essential that the nurse remain nonjudgmental in these situations. The nurse should express concern over the patient's statement and encourage the patient to express thoughts and feelings. If the patient's concerns are caused in part by deviations from required diet, the nurse should investigate possible solutions to fulfill the required dietary needs, be it ordering certain foods, restricting foods, or ritualistic preparation of foods. It may require family member involvement to meet the patient's needs.

It is important to encourage the patient to continue usual and customary religious practices in the hospital. In the perioperative arena, it may be that the patient needs a private moment to pray before induction, or he or she may request that religious medals or beads be with them throughout the procedure. The nurse should attempt to accommodate these wishes if at all possible. If the item interferes with the surgical routine, the nurse can remove the item from the patient after induction and return it at the completion of the procedure.

Some patients may request that a priest or rabbi visit before any procedure. The nurse should attempt to facilitate this request if at all possible. During emergency situations, the support of a clergy may be especially important, not only for the patient, but to offer support and comfort to the family also.

The decision to undergo surgery may involve approval of group elders in a religious community. It is not uncommon for many family and extended family members to gather and support the patient undergoing a procedure. Having a thorough understanding of religious practices is necessary to avoid misunderstandings. For example, shaving of body hair is a violation of religious practices for the Sikh religion of East India.

When language barriers are present, meeting religious needs can prove to be a more challenging situation for the nurse [4]. In some cultures, certain rules and behaviors are instituted before receiving health care services. An understanding of these practices will assist in developing a plan of care individualized to meet the patient's specific needs. In certain situations, the nurse may need to develop strategies to assist the patient and family in the decision to proceed with surgery. Some cultures base all interventions on the zodiac. For example, when trying to convince the patient and family that it would be detrimental to wait until a full moon to perform emergency surgery, the use of tact and understanding is critical [5].

It is also essential for the nurse to understand that folk medicine may play a part in the patient's decision to receive health care services. Some cultures believe in the natural and supernatural world. The rites and rituals of these cultures may impact the Western medical approach to treating certain illnesses directly. It is essential that the nurse receive complete and accurate information from the patient and family on how the patient has been treated before entering the health care system. This is important, because certain home remedies can affect treatment modalities instituted in the hospital setting adversely. For example, certain herbal remedies may be contraindicated when used in conjunction with anesthetic agents [6,7].

The nurse also may encounter a patient and family who believe the illness is God's wish. In these situations, the nurse must work with the patient and family to correct any misconceptions regarding the illness and medical or surgical intervention. It is important to stress the benefit of the health care practices that are being recommended. The nurse must continue to evaluate whether the patient is following the recommended routine. This can be especially challenging in the outpatient setting when the nurse must rely on follow-up conversations to determine compliance [8]. In these situations, it may be best to formulate questions regarding postoperative care that cannot be answered with a simple yes or no answer. Instead, questions should be formulated that would necessitate the patient or family member elaborating on how postoperative care is being performed. Examples of follow-up questions include:

- When you removed the dressing, what did the wound look like? What exactly did you put on the wound?
- Tell me exactly what the patient has had to drink in the last 24 hours?
- Describe for me how the patient did when he or she got out of bed to go to the bathroom.

Questions like these can elicit responses to help the nurse determine if recommended practices are being followed. If the nurse receives responses indicating that herbal teas and concoctions are being administered, or that the patient has not gotten out of bed, because faith healers are administering treatments and performing rituals, this can indicate that the patient and family are mixing Western medicine and cultural rituals. Based on the information given, it may be necessary for the nurse to attempt to re-educate the family.

Spirituality and religion play important roles in the delivery of health care services [9]. Having a full understanding of the religious practices and preferences of the patient and family is necessary to provide for the patient as a whole.

LANGUAGE

Communication is the key ingredient of the nurse–patient relationship. Breaks in communication can lead to misunderstanding, confusion, and error, all of which can lead to a negative outcome. In the perioperative setting, it is imperative that patients have a full understanding of what they will be experiencing. There can be numerous barriers to achieving effective communication. These include, but are not limited to, language barriers, hearing deficit, developmental issues, literacy level, and cultural barriers. The perioperative nurse must assess each individual patient to determine which strategy would work best in each particular situation.

It is important that the nurse begin any new encounter by introducing her/himself to the patient and family. The nurse should exhibit confidence in his or her role and avoid arrogance. If it is appropriate, the nurse should shake hands with the patient and family members. Explain the reason of the visit and explain the sequence of events that will take place. If the first encounter is in the preoperative holding area, explain the assessment, interview by anesthesia provider, admission to the operating room, operative procedure, application of dressings, admission to the perianesthesia care unit, and discharge routine. This will assist the patient and family in understanding the process. It also will help family members understand the time element. For example, many outpatient surgical procedures can be performed and the patient recovered and ready for discharge in as little as 2 to 3 hours, whereas complex inpatient surgical procedures may take as long as 6 hours. Preparing the family in advance will assist in keeping anxiety levels to a minimum. It is also important to review the expectations of the patient and family members.

The nurse should not assume the ethnic and cultural background of the patient. If the patient wants the nurse to know his or her background, he or she will tell the nurse. It is especially important to show respect to all males [10]. In some cultures, the male is considered the head of family, and all decisions go through him, even if it is the wife or child who is undergoing the procedure [11,12]. It is customary in some cultures for children to accompany their parents everywhere. It is important that the children be included in the perioperative experience.

With the diverse population present in the United States today, it is not unusual to encounter patients who either do not speak English or who have English as a second language [12–14]. It is important for the nurse to find ways to communicate effectively so that pre- and postoperative instructions are understood.

There are some strategies to assist the nurse when faced with a culturally sensitive situation [15,16]. Invite the family members to choose where they would like to sit or stand. This allows them to select a distance that is comfortable. Observe how the patient and family interact with others. This will give clues as to what gestures are acceptable and appropriate, such as hand shaking and eye contact. It is important for the nurse to avoid appearing rushed. If nonverbal cues are used in response to questions, it is important to ask for clarification.

For each culture, it is important to learn the proper terms of address. Speak in a positive tone of voice, speaking slowly and clearly. It is extremely important to speak in a normal tone of voice. All too often the nurse will increase the tone and volume when speaking to compensate for the patient's language barrier and poor comprehension [17].

It is important to encourage the patient and family to ask questions. It is helpful if the nurse can learn a few basic words in the patient's native language. This can help break the tension of the situation and put the family at ease. When speaking with the patient and family, avoid professional terms that may have no meaning to them [18]. It is important to explain why certain questions are being asked and what the information will be used for. When giving instructions and information, it is important to repeat the information more than once. It is also beneficial to ask that the information be reiterated back to ensure proper understanding. When prescriptions are given, it is important to review why the medication is needed and what it will do.

When feasible, written instructions should be provided in the patient's native language. This is a great project for nurses to undertake. It provides a chance to work with members of the community. This is also a good opportunity to learn some of the cultural background of each specific culture.

When necessary, the use of an interpreter should be provided to ensure the patient and family have complete understanding of what is happening [19,20]. It is critical that family members not be placed in the position of having to interpret for the patient. This can lead to an uncomfortable situation for both the patient and the family members doing the interpreting. The facility should employ the services of a paid interpreter. Whenever possible, the gender of the interpreter should be the same as that of the patient. The opportunity to be alone with the patient may be difficult because of family practices, but nevertheless, the opportunity should be provided so that sensitive questions may be reviewed in private. It is here that the gender of the interpreter becomes so important. Females may not answer questions or discuss problems in the presence of a male in certain cultures [11,12]. It is also forbidden in some cultures for a male to touch or look at a female who is not in full dress and vice-versa.

Hearing loss can contribute to ineffective communication between the patient and the health care worker. In the perioperative setting, this can lead to the patient not fully understanding the importance of adhering to the preoperative instructions that are reviewed with the patient. Noncompliance with NPO instructions or information concerning which routine medications to take or withhold on the day of surgery can lead to disaster in the operating room. Imagine the potential impact on the surgical patient who continues to take his anticoagulation therapy despite instructions to stop 5 days before surgery; or the severe hypertensive patient who omits his antihypertensive medication because he misunderstood the preoperative instructions. It is not uncommon to find an elderly patient nodding as if in agreement with instructions and information that is being communicated, yet, when asked to reiterate the exchange that has just occurred, the patient is unable to. Patients with hearing deficits often are able to conceal their loss by becoming proficient at lip reading. The nurse must be astute and use keen observation skills to determine if the patient is indeed hiding a hearing loss. It is imperative that written instructions be given to the patient not only preoperatively, but postoperatively also. Again, providing these instructions in the patient's native language is essential to ensure compliance.

When communicating with a patient who is hard of hearing, provide a quiet area, free from distraction and outside noise. Be sure the lighting is adequate. If necessary, provide an interpreter. Determine the patient's preferred method of communication. This could be the use of hearing aids, sign language, lip reading, written communication or a combination of methods. Sit or stand directly in front of the patient and be sure your mouth is visible. Do not chew gum or eat food while communicating and be sure to speak at a comfortable volume. Speak slowly and distinctly; do not exaggerate pronunciation of words. Be sure to maintain eye contact with the patient. It is best to convey the information in as few words as possible. If an interpreter is used, it is essential to speak to the patient, not the interpreter. The interpreter should sit or stand beside the nurse, across from the patient.

When communicating with a hearing impaired patient, it is essential to allocate sufficient time to review the information. The nurse should be astute to recognize nonverbal behaviors that indicate the patient is experiencing anxiety. The patient may be feeling anxious because of his or her hearing disability, and he or she may have concerns on how he or she will be able to get through the upcoming procedure. Offer reassurance and provide a means to maintain communication throughout the patient's stay. It may be that the interpreter accompanies the patient into the operating room and stays through induction and then returns at the end of the procedure to assist in translating to the patient during emergence from anesthesia. Another suggestion is that the nurse and patient develop certain gestures or signals in advance to indicate that the procedure is complete, and everything went according to plan. This can be as simple as tapping the patient's left hand three times or placing an object in the patient's hand. For patients using assistive devices to hear, these should be left in place if at all possible. If they must be removed, be sure they are returned to the patient as soon as feasible, preferably in the operating room, making sure the device is in proper position.

Communicating with the hearing impaired patient is challenging, but through preplanning, the nurse will be able to provide the patient with all the information necessary for a positive surgical experience.

Illiteracy remains a concern for health care workers [19]. Few patients will admit they cannot read or write, but instead try to cover up their deficiency. The patient who is functionally illiterate can read and write at an elementary level. They often will try to cover their inadequacies through other measures. Examples include the patient who refuses to read the consent and just signs, or the patient who quickly places the printed materials aside or states they have forgotten their glasses. The nurse should assess the patient's ability to comprehend the material that is being presented. It is important to maintain that the patient is not stupid, simply uneducated. If the patient is having difficulty understanding, it may be necessary to repeat the information slowly and clearly. Illiterate patients tend to memorize the information given, because they know they will not be able to read it. In these situations, it may be helpful for the perioperative nurse to phone the patient the day before surgery to review the preoperative instructions concerning NPO status, medications, and transportation. If it appears the patient still does not understand, it may be necessary to incorporate the services of a family member.

It is important for the nurse to realize that there may be cultural barriers to communication. What is acceptable to one culture may be offensive to another. It is important for the nurse to have some understanding of what is or is not acceptable in a given situation [21].

In every culture, a person's name plays an important role. The nurse should never assume that it is acceptable to call a patient by their first name, or for the nurse to be addressed on a first name basis. The specific culture, age, and gender of the patient all play an important role in how the patient wishes to be addressed. It is also important to remember that in some cultures, the head of the family will be the person who communicates to the nurse. The nurse must use caution and avoid being judgmental when the man speaks for his wife.

When assessing the patient's illness, it is important to gather as much pertinent information as possible. Ask the patient to describe his or her problem and what he or she believes caused the illness. This may give the nurse clues as to the patient's underlying beliefs. It is important to listen to the patient's understanding of the illness, as this may reveal previous treatment modalities that the patient has used. Obtaining information on herbal treatments, home remedies, or other rituals that have been tried may prove valuable information to avoid potential complications from anesthetic agents [22].

The nurse who has an understanding of the different cultural practices will be able to develop a plan of care that incorporates western medicine with traditional healing practices [23].

ETHNICITY

In today's society, it is crucial for the nurse to develop and implement clinical practice guidelines to improve the delivery of health care services to patients of diverse backgrounds [24]. In the perioperative setting, this may mean delivering services in ways that are different from traditional methods. In some cultures, many family members may accompany the patient. This can cause disruption in how services routinely are delivered in the perioperative setting. Some cultures require all information be communicated to the eldest male in the family, who is the decision maker. Whatever the culture, the perioperative nurse needs to have an understanding of the impact culture plays in the delivery of health care services [25].

It is important for the perioperative nurse to have a clear understanding of his or her own culture and value systems and set aside personal negative opinions of different cultures. It is important not to project one's own views on the patient through verbal and nonverbal communication. Nonverbal cues that could send the wrong message include: touch, facial expression, eye movement, and body posture. Instead, the nurse should incorporate positive communications that combine verbal and nonverbal elements such as humor and warmth.

It is crucial to show respect for the patient and family, regardless of culture [10,26]. Just as every individual is unique, so is every culture. Box 1 identifies guidelines to assist the nurse in relating to patients from different cultures.

In the preoperative area, cultural differences may dictate the type of teaching method used to relay important preoperative information. The surgical consent may present a challenge, as the head of the family or a group of elders may make the decision for surgery. It is important to recognize that

Box 1: Guidelines for relating to patients from different cultures

Assess your personal beliefs surrounding persons from different cultures.

- Review your personal beliefs and past experiences.
- Set aside any values, biases, ideas, and attitudes that are judgmental and may affect care negatively.

Assess communication variables from a cultural perspective.

- Determine the ethnic identity of the patient, including generation in America.
- Use the patient as a source of information when possible.
- Assess cultural factors that may affect your relationship with the patient and respond appropriately.

Plan care based on the communicated needs and cultural background.

- Learn as much as possible about the patient's cultural customs and beliefs.
- Encourage the patient to reveal cultural interpretations of health, illness, and health care.
- Be sensitive to the uniqueness of the patient.
- Identify sources of discrepancy between the patient's and your own concepts of health and illness.
- Communicate at the patient's personal level of functioning.
- Evaluate effectiveness of nursing actions and modify nursing care plan when necessary.

Modify communication approaches to meet cultural needs.

- Be attentive to signs of fear, anxiety, and confusion in patients.
- Respond in a reassuring manner in keeping with the patient's cultural orientation.
- Be aware that in some cultural groups, discussion concerning the patient with others may be offensive and may impede the nursing process.

Understand that respect for the patient and communicated needs are central to the therapeutic relationship.

- Communicate respect by using a kind and attentive approach.
- Learn how listening is communicated in the patient's culture.
- Use appropriate active listening techniques.
- Adopt an attitude of flexibility, respect, and interest to help bridge barriers imposed by culture.

Communicate in a nonthreatening manner.

- Conduct the interview in an unhurried manner.
- Follow acceptable social and cultural amenities.

- Ask general questions during the information-gathering stage.
- Be patient with a respondent who gives information that may seem unrelated to the patient's health problem.
- Develop a trusting relationship by listening carefully, allowing time, and giving the patient your full attention.

Use validating techniques in communication.
- Be alert for feedback that the patient is not understanding.
- Do not assume meaning is interpreted without distortion.

Be considerate of reluctance to talk when the subject involves sexual matters.
- Be aware that in some cultures sexual matters are not discussed freely with members of the opposite sex.

Adopt special approaches when the patient speaks a different language.
- Use a caring tone of voice and facial expression to help alleviate the patient's fears.
- Speak slowly and distinctly, but not loudly.
- Use gestures, pictures, and play-acting to help the patient understand.
- Repeat the message in different ways if necessary.
- Be alert to words the patient seems to understand and use them frequently.
- Keep messages simple and repeat them frequently.
- Avoid using medical terms and abbreviations that the patient may not understand.

Use interpreters to improve communication.
- Ask the interpreter to translate the message, not just the individual words.
- Obtain feedback to confirm understanding.
- Use an interpreter who is culturally sensitive.

From Giger JN, Davidhizar RE. Transcultural nursing: assessment and intervention. St. Louis (MO): Mosby; 1999. p. 34; with permission.

in these situations, the facility policy will dictate who actually will sign the consent.

Removing certain articles or jewelry may interfere with certain cultural practices. If possible, secure the item using tape or another acceptable method. If it must be removed because it interferes with the surgical procedure, determine if it is acceptable to place the article on a different body part. Be sure to document in the nursing record actions taken.

Table 2 identifies cultural behaviors that are relevant to health assessment. It is important for the nurse to have complete understanding so as to practice cultural behaviors that are acceptable to the patient and to avoid behaviors that may be considered off limits.

Table 2
Cultural behaviors relevant to health assessment

Cultural group	Cultural variations (common belief/practice)	Nursing implications
African American	Dialect and slang terms require careful communication to prevent error (ie, bad may mean good).	Question the client's meaning or intent.
Mexican American	Eye behavior is important. An individual who looks at and admires a child without touching the child has given the child the evil eye.	Always touch the child you are examining or admiring.
Native American	Eye contact is considered a sign of disrespect and thus is avoided.	Recognize that the client may be attentive and interested even though eye contact is avoided.
Appalachian	Eye contact is considered impolite or a sign of hostility. Verbal patter may be confusing.	Avoid excessive eye contact. Clarify statements.
American Eskimo	Body language is very important. The individual seldom disagrees publicly with others. Client may nod yes to be polite, even if not in agreement.	Monitor own body language closely as well as client's to detect meaning.
Jewish American	Orthodox Jews consider excess touching, particularly from members of the opposite sex, offensive.	Establish whether client is an Orthodox Jew and avoid excessive touch.
Chinese American	Individual may nod head to indicate yes or shake head to indicate no. Excessive eye contact indicates rudeness. Excessive touch is offensive.	Ask questions carefully and clarify responses. Avoid excessive eye contact and touch.
Haitian American	Touch is used in conversation. Direct eye contact is used to gain attention and respect during communication.	Use direct eye contact when communicating.
East Indian Hindu American	Women avoid eye contact as a sign of respect.	Be aware that men may view eye contact by women as offensive. Avoid eye contact.

Table 2
(continued)

Cultural group	Cultural variations (common belief/practice)	Nursing implications
Phillipino American	Offending people is to be avoided at all costs. Nonverbal behavior is very important.	Monitor nonverbal behaviors of self and client, being sensitive to physical and emotional discomfort or concerns of the client. Use direct eye contact when communicating.
Vietnamese American	Avoidance of eye contact is a sign of respect. The head is considered sacred; it is not polite to pat the head. An upturned palm is offensive in communication	Limit eye contact. Touch the head only when mandated and explain clearly before proceeding to do so. Avoid hand gesturing

From Giger JN, Davidhizar RE. Transcultural nursing: Assessment and intervention. 4th edition. St. Louis (MO): Elsevier; 2004.

SUMMARY

The nurse plays a key role in helping the patient and family understand the perioperative routine. Working with the family to develop adequate means to communicate concerns is instrumental in achieving a positive experience. Identifying with verbal and nonverbal cues when communicating with the patient and family allows the nurse to modify the plan of care to meet individual patient needs. Cultural diversity will continue to be present in society. Establishing an understanding and acceptance of each patient as an individual will help to create an environment where the patient can receive care and treatment in a manner that is culturally acceptable [27].

References

[1] Amerson R. Cultural nursing care: the planning, development, and implementation of a learning experience. J Nurses Staff Dev 2001;17(1):20–4.

[2] Rogers G. Making sense of spirituality in nursing practice—an interactive approach. AORN J 2004;79(5).

[3] Brooks N. Overview of religions. Clin Cornerstone 2004;6(1):7–16.

[4] Odom-Forren J. Cultural competence: a call to action. J Perianesth Nurs 2005;20(2): 79–81.

[5] Peters-Engl C, Frank W, Kerschbaum F, et al. Lunar phases—statistical analysis. Breast Cancer Res Treat 2001;70(2):131–5.

[6] Wolfe K. Herbal remedies. Available at: www.healthpedia.com/herbal-remedies. Accessed October 14, 2005.

[7] Reuters. Herbal remedies cause problems in surgery. Available at: www.Rense.com. Accessed October 14, 2005.

[8] Burden N, Quinn D, O'Brien D. Ambulatory surgical nursing. 2nd edition. St. Louis (MO): Eslevier; 2000.

[9] O'Brien ME. Spirituality in nursing: standing on holy ground. 2nd edition. Sudbury (MA): Jones & Bartlett; 2003.

[10] Anderson R. R.T.S. and cultural competency: quality care hinges on respect, knowledge. ARST-Scanner 2000;32(9):6–8.

[11] Cioffi J. Caring for women from culturally diverse backgrounds: midwives' experiences. J Midwifery Womens Health 2004;49(5):437–42.

[12] Blackford J, Street A. Cultural conflict: the impact of western feminism(s) on nurses caring for women of non-English speaking background. J Clin Nurs 2002;11:664–71.

[13] Dawes BS. Communicating nursing care and crossing language barriers. AORN J 2001;73(5):982.

[14] Wood BA. Caring for a limited-English proficient patient. AORN J 2002;75(5):919–20.

[15] Giger JN, Davidhizar RE. Transcultural nursing: assessment and intervention. 4th edition. St. Louis (MO): Elsevier; 2004.

[16] Boi S. Nurses experiences in caring for patients from different cultural backgrounds. NT Research 2000;5(5):382–90.

[17] Byrne M. Instructional bias—awareness and reduction in perioperative education. AORN J 2002;75(4):808–16.

[18] Ayonride O. Importance of cultural sensitivity in therapeutic transactions: considerations for healthcare providers. Disease Management and Health Outcomes 2003;11(4):233–48.

[19] Dreger V, Tremback T. Optimize patient health by treating literacy and language barriers. AORN J 2002;75(2):280–93.

[20] Collins AS, Gullette D, Schnepf M. Break through language barriers. Nurs Manage 35(8):34–8.

[21] Campinha-Bacote J. Many faces: addressing diversity in healthcare. Journal of Issues in Nursing 2003;8(1):2.

[22] Flowers L. Giving culturally competent care another element in patient safety. OR Manager 2005;21(2):1–18.

[23] Schroeter K. Ethics in perioperative practice—principles and applications. AORN J 2002;75(4):818–24.

[24] American Nurses Association. ANA position statement: ethics and human rights position statements. Cultural diversity in nursing practice. Council on Cultural Diversity in Nursing Practice, Congress on Nursing. Silver Spring (MD): American Nurses Association; 1991.

[25] Steefel L. When culture meets the OR. Nurs Spectr 2000;12(17):4–5.

[26] Andersson M, Mendes IA, Trevizan MA. Universal and culturally dependent issues in healthcare ethics. Med Law 2002;21(1):77–85.

[27] Chin JL. Culturally competent health care. Public Health Rep 2000;115(1):25–33.

[28] Athar S. Information for health care providers when dealing with a Muslim patient. Available at: http://islam_usa.com/e40.html. Accessed October 14, 2005.

Nurs Clin N Am 41 (2006) 249–263

NURSING CLINICS
OF NORTH AMERICA

SEVIER
UNDERS

Bariatric Surgery Risks, Benefits, and Care of the Morbidly Obese

Tracy Martinez Owens, RN, BSN

Wittgrove Bariatric Center, Scripps Memorial Hospital,
9438 Genesee Avenue, Suite 328, La Jolla, CA 92037, USA

The American Society for Bariatric Surgery defines *morbid obesity* as a life-long, progressive, life-threatening, genetically related, costly, multifactorial disease of excess fat storage with multiple comorbidities. Obesity satisfies the definition of morbid obesity when it reaches the point of significant risk for obesity-related comorbidities. These significant comorbidities often result in either significant physical disability or even death [1]. Obesity results from excessive accumulation of fat that exceeds the body skeletal and physical standards. Morbid obesity is defined as being at least 100 lb heavier than ideal body weight, or a body mass index (BMI) of 40. BMI is calculated as weight in kilograms divided by the height in meters squared. This article focuses on the causes, treatment, and perioperative nursing care of patients who are morbidly obese.

OBESITY IS THE GREATEST EMERGING PUBLIC HEALTH CRISIS

Worldwide obesity affects more than 250 million individuals. Based on the US Census Bureau statistics for the year 2000, 129.6 million (64.5%) Americans older than 20 years are overweight [1,2]. Approximately 10 million people qualify as morbidly obese, with a BMI more than 40 [1]. Some of the most alarming statistics are in children, predicting an even graver future. The proportion of obese and overweight children and adolescents in the United States nearly doubled in the 1980s alone, and the numbers continue to rise. This trend is likely to increase; more than 25% of children between the age of 2 and 19 years surveyed in 1999 to 2000 were overweight or obese [3,4]. Morbid obesity, also called *clinically severe obesity*, is a medical disease that describes an individual who is 100 lb heavier than ideal body weight or a BMI of 40 or more [5,6]. Morbid obesity is a chronic disease, meaning its symptoms worsen

E-mail address: towensrn@lapbypass.com

0029-6465/06/$ – see front matter
doi:10.1016/j.cnur.2006.01.008

over an extended period. The more common comorbidities associated with morbid obesity are

- Type 2 diabetes mellitus
- Obstructive sleep apnea (OSA)
- Gastroesophageal reflux disease (GERD)
- Osteoarthritis of the weight-bearing joints

Type 2 Diabetes Mellitus

Obese individuals develop a resistance to insulin because of increased adipose tissue. The potential for an individual to develop diabetes doubles for every 20% increase over the desired weight [7,8].

Hypertension

Excess body weight puts stress on the cardiac system, compromising its ability to function properly. Hypertension can increase an individual's risk for stroke and heart and kidney damage. Evidence shows that the age-related lifetime risk for hypertension in men and women ages 45 to 54 years will double as their average BMI increases from 25 to 35 [9].

Obstructive Sleep Apnea

OSA is an often-undiagnosed life-threatening comorbidity. OSA occurs when the accumulation of excess soft tissue in the posterior aspect of the throat causes the airway to close and breathing to stop. These deposits in the tongue and neck cause intermittent obstruction [10].

Gastroesophageal Reflux Disease

Excess abdominal weight causes digestive acid to be pushed up into the esophagus, resulting in complaints of heartburn. Without appropriate medical attention, Barrett's esophagus may occur. Patients often complain of asthma that results from aspiration of gastric acid, especially during sleeping hours. A 5- to 10-year follow-up study that included 16,191 participants showed that an independent relationship exists between obesity, nighttime GERD, and habitual snoring, and the onset of asthma and respiratory symptoms in adults [11]. Another study involving 130 patients showed that people who suffer from GERD experience a worsening of symptoms as their weight increases [12].

Osteoarthritis of the Weight-Bearing Joints

Excess weight placed on joints leads to wear and tear, causing arthritis [13]. Excess weight placed on joints, particularly knees and hips, results in rapid breakdown of the joint cartilage leading to painful inflammation and osteoarthritis. In addition to joint pain, individuals who are morbidly obese often complain of back pain and strain, commonly resulting in disc problems and decreased mobility.

The psychologic impact on those who are morbidly obese is a great burden. Unfortunately many individuals who are morbidly obese have endured a lifetime of loneliness and discrimination. Latner and colleagues [14] conducted a study on children's attitudes toward obesity. They found children as young as 6 years described silhouettes of an obese child as lazy, dirty, stupid, ugly, a cheater, and a liar. The psychologic aspects of this disease are as important as the more publicized major medical comorbid conditions when considering quality of life [15–17].

One of many misunderstandings about those who are morbidly obese is that they are in the upper percentile for psychologic illness. On the contrary, studies of people who were severely overweight before undergoing weight-loss surgery have shown that no single personality type characterizes people who are severely obese. This population does not report greater levels of psychopathy than the average-weight control population [18]. However, depression is high in the population participating in the author's program.

Other common comorbidities that affect quality of life include depression, infertility, lower-extremity venous stasis, stress urinary incontinence, dyslipidemia, deep vein thrombosis (DVT), and pulmonary embolism. Individuals who are morbidly obese are at increased risk for some cancers, including colorectal, breast, ovarian, gallbladder, prostate, endometrial, and uterine. Pseudotumor cerebri is another condition seen in the morbidly obese population because of elevated cerebrospinal fluid pressure. If left untreated, pseudotumor cerebri can cause visual loss [1,18].

In 1991, the National Institutes of Health (NIH) established guidelines for the surgical treatment of patients who are morbidly obese [19]. These guidelines state that surgery is indicated for individuals who have a BMI of 40 or 35 if the patient has significant comorbidities. Also published in this statement is the fact that individuals who are morbidly obese cannot sustain weight loss with nonsurgical diet therapy.

SURGICAL OPTIONS FOR BARIATRIC SURGERY

Occasionally, a procedure will be considered for someone with a BMI of 35 to 39.9 if the patient's obesity-related health conditions have resulted in a medical need for weight reduction and, in the doctor's opinion, surgery seems to be the only way to accomplish the targeted weight loss [18].

Most nonsurgical weight loss programs are based on some combination of diet and behavior modification and regular exercise. However, even the most effective interventions are only so for a small percentage of individuals. Less than 5% of individuals who participate in nonsurgical weight loss programs are estimated to lose a significant amount of weight and maintain that loss for a long period [20]. According to the NIH, most people in these programs regain their weight within 1 year [1]. Patients who are morbidly obese have an even harder time sustaining weight loss. Serious health risks have been identified for people who move from diet to diet, subjecting their bodies to a severe and continuing cycle of weight loss and gain known as *yo-yo dieting.*

Each time an individual diets on a very low-calorie diet without adequate protein intake, the body loses muscle mass. Besides the health risk, the loss of muscle mass decreases the metabolic rate, thereby making it almost impossible to maintain any weight loss.

Morbid obesity is a complex, multifactorial chronic disease. Weight-loss surgery, when compared with other interventions, has provided the longest period of sustained weight loss in patients for whom all other therapies have failed [18]. Americans spend $33 billion annually on weight-loss products and services, including low-calorie foods, artificially sweetened products, and commercial weight-loss centers [1,21]. Despite these efforts, obesity among adults has increased by nearly 60% since 1991 [3,4].

For many patients, the risk for death from not undergoing the surgery is greater than the risks from possible surgical complications. This risk is the key reason that, in 2004, approximately 140,600 weight-loss surgical procedures were performed, and the same reason an estimated 173,000 people will seek the benefits of bariatric surgery in 2005 [22]. Patients who have undergone the procedure and are benefiting from its results report improvements in

- Quality of life
- Social interactions
- Psychologic well-being
- Employment opportunities
- Economic condition

HISTORY

The first bariatric procedures occurred in the 1950s [23]. Kremen and colleagues successfully performed a jejuno-ileal bypass (JIB) in 1954. In 1952, Victor Henriksson of Gothenberg, Sweden, performed a similar procedure for morbid obesity. Dr. Richard Varco of the University of Minnesota independently performed a JIB at the University of Minnesota Hospitals around the same time Kremen and colleagues performed their operation. Two variants were subsequently developed: the *end-to-side* in 1969 and the *end-to end* in 1973 [23]. In both instances an extensive length of small intestine was bypassed, not excised, excluding it from the alimentary stream [23]. A modern improvement of the JIB is biliopancreatic diversion (BPD), developed by Professor Nicola Scopinaro and colleagues of the University of Genoa in 1996 [23].

Gastric bypass (RGB) was developed by Dr. Edward E. Mason of the University of Iowa in 1967. In 1988, Hess developed a hybrid operation, the *duodenal switch*. This procedure was originally designed for patients who had bile reflux gastritis, and consists of a suprapapillary Roux-en-Y duodenojejunostomy with stomach volume reduction. This technique, first presented by Hess in 1992, is now known as biliopancreatic diversion with duodenal switch (BPDDS) [23].

In 1990, Dr. Kuzmak developed an ingenious devise, the inflatable band with a balloon as its lining, which became the current gastric banding procedure [23,24]. Finally, the first laparoscopic gastric bypass was performed in 1993 by Dr. Alan C. Wittgrove. Today most bariatric procedures are performed laparoscopically, reducing the risk for wound infection and incisional hernia and decreasing hospital stay.

PROCEDURES
Three basic categories of bariatric surgery are performed today: restrictive, malabsorptive, and combination procedures.

Restrictive Procedures
Restrictive procedures restrict the amount of food that can be ingested, therefore limiting the quantity of food consumed. Restrictive procedures do not interfere with absorption of food, vitamins, or nutrients.

The most common restrictive procedure today is *adjustable gastric banding* [25]. This procedure is commonly performed laparoscopically, and is called *laparoscopic adjustable gastric banding* (LAGB) (Fig. 1). Gastric banding is performed by placing a silastic band around the uppermost part of the stomach. The band creates a small pouch that regulates the amount of food consumed. The band is periodically tightened on an individual basis through a reservoir port that is accessible through the subcutaneous tissue. The port is accessible using a Huber needle. Box 1 lists the advantages, disadvantages, and risks of LAGB.

Malabsorptive Procedures
Two of the more common malabsorptive procedures of today are the BPD (Fig. 2) and the BPDDS (Fig. 3).

BPD is less commonly performed than the more recent modification, the duodenal switch [23]. The BPD involves a subtotal gastrectomy that leaves a much larger gastric pouch compared with the Roux-en-Y gastric bypass (RYGB) or the adjustable gastric band. The small bowel is divided 250 cm

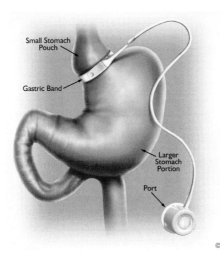

Fig. 1. Adjustable gastric band. (Courtesy of Ethicon Endo-Surgery [copyright owner, all rights reserved]; with permission.)

Box 1: Advantages, disadvantages, and risks of adjustable gastric banding

Advantages

- Restricts the amount of food that can be consumed at a meal, therefore limiting calories consumed
- Food consumed passes through the digestive tract in the usual order, allowing it to be fully absorbed into the body without any malabsorption
- Band can be adjusted to increase or decrease restriction
- Band is removable

Disadvantages

- May not provide a sense of satiety (ie, feeling full but not satisfied) and therefore may lead to snacking or "grazing" throughout the day
- Less weight loss than other bariatric surgeries. In a United States study the mean weight loss at 3 years following surgery was only 36.2% to 47.5% excess body weight in meta-analysis review of over 1800 patients [26,27]

Risks

- Gastric perforation or tearing in the stomach wall may require additional operation
- Access port leakage or twisting may require additional operation
- Nausea and vomiting
- Outlet obstruction
- Pouch dilatation
- Band migration/slippage
- Gastric wall ulceration or erosion

proximal to the ileocecal valve and connected directly to the gastric pouch, producing a gastroileostomy. The remaining proximal limb (biliopancreatic conduit) is then anastomosed to the side of the distal ileum 50 cm proximal to the ileocecal valve. In this procedure, the distal stomach, duodenum, and entire jejunum are bypassed, leaving only a 50-cm distal ileum common channel for nutrients to mix with pancreatic and biliary secretions.

The BPDDS is a variation of the BPD that preserves the first portion of the duodenum and pylorus. In this procedure, a vertical, subtotal gastrectomy is performed and the duodenum is divided several centimeters beyond the pylorus. The distal small bowel is connected to the duodenal stump, producing a 75- to 100-cm ileal-duodenal common channel. The other end of the duodenum is closed and the remaining small bowel is connected onto the enteral limb at about 75 to 100 cm from the ileocecal valve. Box 2 lists the advantages, disadvantages, and risks of malabsorptive procedures.

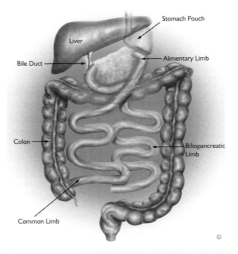

Fig. 2. Biliopancreatic diversion. (Courtesy of Ethicon Endo-Surgery [copyright owner, all rights reserved]; with permission.)

Combination or Hybrid Procedure

The RYGB (Fig. 4) is the most commonly performed and accepted bypass procedure. RYGB is commonly referred to as the "gold standard" procedure of weight-loss procedures and is the most frequently performed procedure in the United States [22]. It involves forming a 10- to 30-mL proximal gastric pouch by surgically separating or stapling the stomach across the fundus.

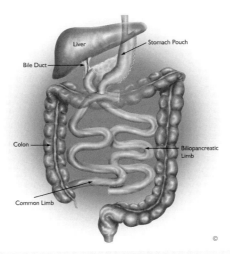

Fig. 3. Duodenal switch. (Courtesy of Ethicon Endo-Surgery [copyright owner, all rights reserved]; with permission.)

Box 2: Advantages, disadvantages, and risks of malabsorptive procedures

Advantages

- May produce greater weight loss because they provide the greatest amount of malabsorption
- Some patients prefer to be able to consume larger amounts of food because of the larger gastric pouch (compared with restrictive or combination procedures)
- In the meta-analysis review, patients who underwent BPD and duodenal switch surgery experienced a mean weight loss of 70.12% [27]

Disadvantages

- Gastrointestinal leak at the anastomotic sight may occur
- Changes to the intestinal absorption will increase chances for gallbladder disease
- Patients commonly suffer from frequent, liquid, malodorous stool (steatorrhea) caused by the malabsorptive component of the operation
- Abdominal bloating and gas may occur. Lifelong monitoring for protein malnutrition, anemia, and bone disease, and lifelong vitamin supplementation are recommended

Risks

- Vitamin deficiencies of fat-soluble vitamins (A, D, E, and K) may occur even with minimal noncompliance
- Rerouting of the bile and digestive juices can lead to intestinal irritation and ulcer formation
- Menstruating women may be more prone to anemia caused by malabsorption of vitamin B_{12} and iron
- Decreased absorption of calcium may also trigger osteoporosis and metabolic bone disease
- RGB and BPD operations may also cause *dumping syndrome*, in which stomach contents move too rapidly through the small intestine. Symptoms include nausea, weakness, sweating, faintness, and sometimes diarrhea after eating

Outflow from the pouch is created by performing a narrow (10- to 12-mm) gastrojejunostomy. The proximal end of jejunum is then anastomosed 75 to 150 cm below the gastrojejunostomy. *Roux-en-Y* refers to the Y-shaped section of the small intestine created by the surgery. The Y is created at the point where the biliopancreatic conduit and the Roux limb are connected. Bypass refers to the exclusion or bypassing of the distal stomach, duodenum, and proximal jejunum [28]. RYGB is endorsed by the NIH 1991 Consensus Development Panel [4] and may be performed with an open incision or laparoscopically. A distal RYGB adds a malabsorptive component by making the common limb shorter, thereby producing malabsorption. The proximal end of the jejunum

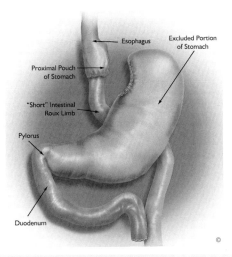

Fig. 4. Gastric bypass Roux-en-Y. (Courtesy of Ethicon Endo-Surgery [copyright owner, all rights reserved]; with permission.)

is anastomosed closer to the cecum, thus allowing a shorter common channel. Box 3 lists the advantages, disadvantages, and risks of RYGB.

BENEFITS OF BARIATRIC SURGERY

The benefit of bariatric surgery, aside from weight loss, is that it resolves or greatly improves obesity-related comorbidities. This health improvement provides a greater quality of life and increases lifespan. The prevalence of type 2 diabetes mellitus, hypertension, OSA, heart disease, and stroke accounts for more than 2.5 million deaths worldwide each year [30]. *JAMA* reported that years of lost life caused by morbid obesity were approximately 12 years fewer for a 25-year-old morbidly obese man [31]. Obesity surgery is currently the only modality that shows long-term weight loss. Conventional diets do not maintain sustainable weight loss for those who are morbidly obese.

According to a meta-analysis (an in-depth study reviewing multiple procedures performed at academic and private practice centers), a study of 1846 patients who had type 2 diabetes mellitus showed that 1417 experienced complete resolution. Another study reported improvement or resolution in diabetes in 414 out of 485 patients, including improvements in glycosylated hemoglobin (HgbA₁c), fasting glucose, and fasting insulin. A 47.9% resolution of type 2 diabetes mellitus occurred in patients who underwent gastric banding, an 83.7% resolution in those who underwent RYGB, and a 98.9% resolution in those who underwent BPD or duodenal switch [27].

This vast study also reported substantial improvements (70% or more) in hyperlipidemia after all bariatric procedures. The best improvement in hyperlipidemia (99%) was seen in the BPD or duodenal switch procedures. RYGB

Box 3: Advantages, disadvantages, and risks of Roux-en-Y gastric bypass

Advantages

- The average excess weight loss is generally higher in patients who are compliant with prescribed regimens than in those undergoing purely restrictive procedures
- One year after surgery, weight loss can average 77% of excess body weight [29]
- Studies show that after 10 to 14 years, patients maintain 60% of excess body weight loss
- In 2000, a study of 500 patients showed that 96% of certain associated health conditions (back pain, sleep apnea, high blood pressure, diabetes, and depression) improved or resolved [29]
- Dumping syndrome can occur as the result of rapid emptying of stomach contents into the small intestine, sometimes triggered when too much sugar or large amounts of food are consumed. Symptoms include nausea, weakness, sweating, faintness, and occasionally diarrhea after eating. Although some patients may see this as a negative, others feel it is an advantage because it deters them from ingesting sweets

Disadvantages

- In some cases, the effectiveness of the procedure may be reduced if the stomach pouch initially created has a capacity greater than 15–30 ml or if the stomach pouch expands as a result of overeating.

Risks

- Gastrointestinal leak at the gastrojejunostomy or enteroenterostomy anastomotic sites may occur
- Because the duodenum is bypassed, poor absorption of iron and calcium can result in the lowering of total body iron and a predisposition to iron deficiency anemia in patients who are not compliant with vitamin and mineral supplementation. Women should be aware of the potential for heightened bone calcium loss
- Chronic anemia and neurologic deficiencies can occur from vitamin B_{12} deficiency; supplementation is necessary

procedures resulted in a 96% reduction in hyperlipidemia, and gastric banding in a 58.9% decrease [27]. In 4805 patients who had preoperative hypertension, the hypertension improved after bariatric surgery 61.7% of the time.

OSA is prevalent in 60% of patients who have clinically significant obesity [32]. The best treatment for OSA in individuals who are morbidly obese is weight loss, with a cure rate of nearly 100% [33,34].

After RYGB and the gastric banding procedures, acid from the stomach can no longer reach the proximal stomach pouch or esophagus, therefore preventing reflux. Patients report immediate improvement in gastric reflux [29]. Asthma, when secondary to reflux, is also markedly improved.

As seen in Table 1, A. C. Wittgrove showed a marked improvement or resolution (96%) of major comorbidities in 500 patients who underwent LPGB. In this study, all of these comorbidities were graded for significance pre- and postoperatively [29].

PERIOPERATIVE NURSING CARE
Psychologic Support
Expressing sincere empathy for patients who are morbidly obese and showing an understanding of the disease and the discrimination these individuals endure may be the most important aspect of nursing care [5,35].

Morbid obesity is a disease with a strong genetic predisposition. Studies indicate that up to 70% of the variability in human body weight may be accounted for by genetic factors [36]. Often society, including medical personnel, believes that if individuals ate less and exercised more, they could control their weight.

In a survey of nursing attitudes toward people who are obese, nurses reported beliefs that these individuals most likely have issues with anger, are lazy, and are overindulgent [37]. In another study, the persistence of a strong negative evaluation of patients who are obese and the perception that individuals who are overweight are bad and lazy were found in a group of health care professionals specializing in the treatment of obesity [38].

The NIH Consensus Development Statement in 1991 [19] stated that individuals who are morbidly obese cannot sustain weight loss long-term. However, a strong genetic predisposition contributes to becoming morbidly obese. Twin studies show that two thirds of the variation in body weight can be attributed to genetic factors [39].

Empathy training should be mandatory for hospital personnel interfacing with patients who are overweight. Nurses should be comfortable conveying

Table 1
Resolution of comorbidities in 500 patients who underwent laparoscopic gastric bypass followed out to 60 months

Condition	Preoperatively	Postoperatively
GERD	269	4
Hypercholesterol	275	8
Hypertriglyceride	158	1
Diabetes	85	1
Glucose intolerance	50	0
Stress incontinence	201	6
Sleep apnea	225	5
Hypertension	118	10
Arthritis (symptomatic)	371	36
Total	1752	71

Abbreviation: GERD, gastroesophageal reflux disease.
  Data from Ethicon Endo-Surgery (copyright owner, all rights reserved).

empathy and their understanding of the negative psychologic impact morbid obesity causes. Simply making eye contact, touching the patient's arm, and being nonjudgmental can make an enormous emotional difference to this patient population. Nurses often believe that taking care of patients who are obese will be extremely difficult after bariatric surgery. On the contrary, most patients who are morbidly obese try to be too independent because they do not want to hurt the nurses as a result of their size and do not want to draw more attention to their obesity.

Nursing care after bariatric surgery (open or laparoscopic) entails all the routine postoperative assessment that a prudent skilled nurse would perform on any patient who underwent abdominal surgery. However, the nurse must carefully review each patient's history. The comorbidities are the potential complications that need diligent assessment postoperatively [35]. Recognizing the comorbidities is essential in reducing the risk for postoperative complications.

Postoperative respiratory assessment of the patient who is morbidly obese is extremely important. Severe obesity causes decreased ventilation because abdominal fat decreases the movement of the diaphragm, and excess adipose tissue in or around the thorax reduces thoracic expansion. Hypoventilation leads to hypercarbia, decreased oxygen saturation, and daytime somnolence [40]. Respiratory status is compromised by general anesthesia and narcotic administration. If a patient-controlled analgesia is used, close observation is necessary. If a patient experiences sleep apnea, the surgeon may order postoperative continuous positive-airway pressure. Some surgeons are concerned about the pressurized oxygen putting stress on the anastomosis in patients who underwent gastric bypass, BPD, and duodenal switch. Close postoperative observation with pulse oximetry and apnea monitoring is necessary.

Patients who are overweight should be positioned with the head of the bed elevated to 30% to maximize lung expansion. Incentive spirometry should be monitored for continued use in the hospital and should be continued at home to decrease the risk for atelectasis or pneumonia. Early and frequent ambulation also prevents respiratory complications.

Vigilant surveillance of signs and symptoms of surgical complications can have an enormous impact on overall outcome. Regardless of open or laparoscopic approach, anastomotic leaks can be fatal if not recognized early. Although the anastomoses are often tested for leaks intraoperatively with saline or methylene blue dye, leaks can occur when pressure infusion is administered. Symptoms of an anastomotic leak can be overt or subtle. Symptoms can range from abdominal tenderness, left shoulder pain, tachycardia, decreased urine output, fever, elevated white blood cell counts, and oxygen desaturation, to a patient "not looking right" or complaining of a sense of impending doom. When the clinical assessment is known, the surgeon must be notified immediately.

Postoperative leaks may be managed through (1) re-exploration (when the patient is stable and has symptoms of peritonitis or when the patient is hemodynamically unstable), (2) repair of the anastomotic leak, or (3) placement of an abdominal drain by the interventional radiologist (if a patient has a controlled or contained leak or abscess).

Patients who are obese are at greater risk for DVT in the lower extremities than patients who are normal-weighted. Prophylactic measures are necessary to minimize risk. Prophylactic interventions include administration of low molecular weight anticoagulant preoperatively and daily during the hospital stay. Other preventative measures include sequential compression stockings during surgery and during hospital stay, and early and frequent ambulation. Patients should be educated on the importance of continued ambulation and activity for continued prevention.

Patients at higher risk for DVT and pulmonary embolism (PE) are those who have a history of thromboembolism. Some surgeons will consider placement of a vena cava filter before surgery for the higher-risk patient.

The importance of skin care and decubitus prevention is often misunderstood or minimized. Proper padding of pressure areas should be initiated and documented in the operating room. Some health care workers believe that because patients who are obese have "extra padding," they don't need padding protection. Nothing could be further from the truth. Patients who are morbidly obese are at greater risk for skin breakdown and infection because of excess weight on bony prominences and less blood supply to the distal subcutaneous tissue [41]. If a patient has diabetes, the risk is greater. Early ambulation, proper hydration, and thorough skin assessment help reduce the risk for skin breakdown and infection.

SUMMARY

Bariatric surgery is a unique field in which one operation can cure an individual's medical diseases (comorbidities) caused by obesity. These procedures require a well-trained, highly skilled open or laparoscopic surgeon working within a multidisciplinary team. It is also prudent to include well-trained nurses who are responsible for postoperative care of patients who are overweight. Perioperative and medical/surgical nurse managers should consider providing ongoing education for the nurses responsible for the care of patients who are overweight. Nursing competencies should also be considered because of the medical, psychologic, and surgical uniqueness of this patient population. Most health care providers believe that patients who are overweight are among the most rewarding individuals to care for, including this author.

Further readings

Caro JF. Clinical review 26: insulin resistance in obese and nonobese men. J Clin Endocrinol Metab 1991;73:691–5.

Centers for Disease Control and Prevention (CDC). Obesity continues to climb in 1999 among American adults; Obesity Trends. Available at: http://www.edu.gov/needphp/dmpa/obesity/trend/prev_char.html. Accessed September 2005.

Cunning H, Mayer J. Obesity—its possible effects on college admissions. N Engl J Med 1966;275:1172–4.

Pories WJ, MacDonald KG Jr, Flickinger EG, et al. Is type II diabetes mellitus (NIDDM) a surgical disease? Ann Surg 1992;215:633–43.
Stunkard AJ, Wadden TA. Psychological aspects of severe obesity. Am J Clin Nutr 1992;55 (2 Suppl):524S–32S.
Yanovski JA, Yanovski SZ. Recent advances in basic obesity research. JAMA 1999;282: 1504–6.

References

[1] Weight-control Information Network. Statistics related to overweight and obesity. Available at: http://www.niddk.nih.gov/statistics/index.htm#preval. Accessed November 2005.

[2] Flegal KM, et al. Prevalence and trends in obesity among US adults, 1999–2000. JAMA 2002;288:1723–7.

[3] Ogden CI, Flegal KM, Carroll D, et al. Prevalence and trends in overweight among US children and adolescents, 1999–2000. JAMA 2002;288:1728–32.

[4] Freedman DS, Khan LK, Serdula MK, et al. Trends and correlates of class 3 obesity in the United States from 1990 through 2000. JAMA 2002;288:1758–61.

[5] AORN. Bariatric surgery guideline. Standards, recommended practices, and guidelines. Denver (CO): The Association; 2005. p. 55–73.

[6] Fields SD, Strano-Paul L. Obesity, an issue of clinics in geriatric medicine. Philadelphia: Saunders; 2005.

[7] Peters-Harmel A, Mathur R. Davidson's diabetes mellitus. 5th edition. Philadelphia: Saunders; 2004.

[8] Bailes BK. Diabetes mellitus and its chronic complications. AORN J 2002;76(2):265–82.

[9] Presutti R, Gorman R, Swain J. Primary care perspective in bariatric surgery. Mayo Clin Proc 2004;79(9):1158–66.

[10] Billington CJ. Measurement of sleep apnea during obesity treatment. Obes Res 2002;10(Suppl 1):38S–41S.

[11] Gunnbjornsdottir MI, Omenaas E, Gislason T, et al. Obesity and nocturnal gastro-oesophageal reflux are related to onset of asthma and respiratory symptoms. Eur Respir J 2004;24: 116–21.

[12] Smith SC, Edwards CB, Goodman GN. Symptomatic and clinical improvement in morbidly obese patients with gastroesophageal reflux disease following Roux-en-Y gastric bypass. Obes Surg 1997;7:479–84.

[13] Hinton R, Moody RL, Davis AW, et al. Osteoarthritis: diagnosis and therapeutic considerations. Am Fam Physician 2002;65(5):841–8.

[14] Latner JD, Stunkard AJ, Wilson GT. Stigmatized students: age, sex, and ethnicity effects in the stigmatization of obesity. Obes Res 2005;13:1226–31.

[15] Eaton DK, Lowry R, Brener ND, et al. Associations of body mass index and perceived weight with suicide ideation and suicide attempts among US high school students. Arch Pediatr Adolesc Med 2005;159(6):513–9.

[16] Zametkin AJ, Zoon CK, Klein HW, et al. Psychiatric aspects of child and adolescent obesity: a review of the past 10 years. J Am Acad Child Adolesc Psychiatry 2004;43(2):134–50, 151–3.

[17] Davison KK, Birch LL. Lean and weight stable: behavioral predictors and psychological correlates. Obes Res 2004;12:1085–93.

[18] Society of Bariatric Surgery. Rationale for the surgical treatment of morbid obesity. Available at: http://www.asbs.org/html/ration.html. Accessed November 2005.

[19] National Institute of Health (NIH). Consensus Development Conference Statement: gastrointestinal surgery for severe obesity. Available at: http://www.consensus.nih.gov/1991/1991GISurgeryObesity084html.htm. Accessed November 2005.

[20] American Society for Bariatric Surgery (ASBS). Surgery for morbid obesity: what patients should know. Toronto: FD–Communications Inc.; 2000.

[21] Scott JR. What are the costs and health expenses of being obese? Available at: http://www.weightloss.about.com/od/obesityhealth/a/bl_costs.htm. Accessed November 2005.

[22] Buchwald H, Williams SE. Bariatric surgery worldwide 2003. Obes Surg 2004;14(9):1157–64.

[23] MacGregor A. The story of surgery for obesity: Kremer, Linner, and other early pioneers. Available at: http://www.asbs.org/html/story/chapter1.html. Accessed November 2005.

[24] Deitel M, Shikora SA. The development of the surgical treatment of morbid obesity. J Am Coll Nutr 2002;21:365–71.

[25] Ferraro DR. Laparoscopic adjustable gastric banding for morbid obesity. AORN J 2003;77(5):923–40.

[26] Inamed Health. Bioenterics® Lap-Band® Adjustable Gastric Banding System, P/N 94800 Rev. J, 10/02. Instructions for use.

[27] Buchwald H, Avidor Y, Braunwald E, et al. Bariatric surgery: a systematic review and meta-analysis. JAMA 2004;292(14):1724–37.

[28] Barrow CJ. Roux-en-Y gastric bypass for morbid obesity. AORN J 2002;76(4):590, 593–604.

[29] Wittgrove AC, Clark GW. Laparoscopic gastric bypass, Roux-en-Y- 500 patients: techniques and results, with 3–60 month follow-up. Obes Surg 2000;10(3):233–9.

[30] World Health Organization. World Health Report 2002. Available at: http://www.iotf.org. Accessed November 2005.

[31] Fontaine KR, Redden DT, Wang C, et al. Years of life lost due to obesity. JAMA 2003;289:187–93.

[32] Serafini FM, MacDowell Anderson W, Rosemurgy AS, et al. Clinical predictors of sleep apnea in patients undergoing bariatric surgery. Obes Surg 2001;11:28–31.

[33] Dhabuwala A, Cannan RJ, Stubbs RS. Improvement in co-morbidities following weight loss from gastric bypass surgery. Obes Surg 2000;10(5):428–35.

[34] Rasheid S, Banasiak M, Gallagher SF, et al. Gastric bypass is an effective treatment for obstructive sleep apnea in patients with clinically significant obesity. Obes Surg 2003;13(1):58–61.

[35] Graling P, Elariny H. Perioperative care of the patient with morbid obesity. AORN J 2003;77(4):802–5, 808–19.

[36] Oken E, Gillman MW. Fetal origins of obesity. Obes Res 2003;11:496–506.

[37] Maroney D, Golub S. Nurses' attitudes toward obese persons and certain ethnic groups. Percept Mot Skills 1992;75(2):387–91.

[38] Teachman BA, Gapinski KD, Brownell KD, et al. Demonstrations of implicit anti-fat bias: the impact of providing casual information and evoking empathy. Health Psychol 2003;22:68–78.

[39] Stunkard AJ, Foch TT, Hrubec Z. A twin study of human obesity. JAMA 1986;256(1):51–4.

[40] Kessler R, Chaouat A, Schinkewitch P, et al. The obesity-hypoventilation syndrome revisited; a prospective study of 34 consecutive cases. Chest 2001;120(2):369–76.

[41] Gruendemann BJ, Mangum SS. Infection prevention in surgical settings. Philadelphia: Saunders; 2001.

Nurs Clin N Am 41 (2006) 265–298

NURSING CLINICS
OF NORTH AMERICA

Unique Concerns of the Pediatric Surgical Patient: Pre-, Intra-, and Postoperatively

Dolly Ireland, MSN, RN, CAPA, CPN[a,b]

[a]Crittenton Hospital Medical Center, 1101 West University Drive, Rochester, MI 48307, USA
[b]Oakland Community College, Highland Lakes, Waterford, MI, USA

This article focuses on the unique concerns of pediatric surgical patients and emphasizes preparation of the family as an integrated unit. The statement from older standards of the American Nurses' Association that "children have the right to be treated with dignity and respect" [1] remains a valid challenge for nurses caring for these patients.

Pediatric patients are not "miniature adults," although the goals and standards of care remain the same as for adults. The surgical problems particular to children from birth to postpuberty are not limited to one area of the body or any one surgical specialty. Effective and developmentally appropriate preparation; thorough assessment of preoperative and postoperative needs; and adequate planning, implementation, and delivery of care safely return the pediatric patient to the preanesthesia state [2].

The perioperative/perianesthesia nurse cares for the child and must also maintain the integrity of the family unit. The nurse assists parents through this educational process by providing them with the necessary information to make informed decisions and offering emotional support to their children.

PRE- THROUGH POSTOPERATIVE PHASES

Caring for a child undergoing surgery requires a coordinated team effort. Three basic phases comprise the perioperative care of the pediatric surgical patient: (1) the physiologic and psychologic preparation of the child and family; (2) the safe and efficient management of the child's surgery/anesthesia in the operating room; and (3) the careful management of the child's immediate postoperative care to minimize complications.

The preoperative or preanesthesia phase is the period before the patient undergoes surgery and anesthesia. Interviews are conducted with the child, if appropriate, and the parents or caregivers who are present. The nurse assesses

E-mail addresses: direland@crittenton.com; idolly@wowway.com

0029-6465/06/$ – see front matter
doi:10.1016/j.cnur.2006.01.007

the pediatric patient's developmental level, psychosocial level, admission vital signs, and medical history and laboratory values, if ordered.

The intraoperative phase is the period spent in the operating room where the procedure is performed while safe, appropriate anesthesia is continually monitored.

The postanesthesia phase I is the period spent in the postanesthesia care unit (PACU) when the child is emerging from a totally anesthetized state; requires continual monitoring and vigilance for adequate respiratory and cardiac function; and has the potential for acute intervention and nursing care.

During the postanesthesia phase II, the child transitions from an anesthetized state to one requiring less acute intervention. The child is with the parents and is being prepared for discharge or transfer to the pediatric unit, depending on the procedure and the condition of the child.

CHARACTERISTICS OF THE PEDIATRIC SURGICAL POPULATION

Children of all ages may be recipients of surgical care. Because of the unique needs of children, parents are also indirect recipients of care. A delicate balance exists among the child, the family, and the nurse (the healing triangle [3]). All three interact to aid in the healing process. The nurse assesses the physical condition, developmental levels, behavioral reactions, and learning readiness and interprets verbal and nonverbal cues. The parents learn about the disease process and the surgical and discharge process, and help interpret the child's emotional responses. The child learns about these processes out of interest, curiosity, and a desire to maintain some control.

The age of pediatric patients varies from neonates to age 18, and the characteristics of the population are very diverse. Children can undergo invasive procedures or surgery in various practice settings. Specialists in all fields develop the necessary skills and knowledge to perform pediatric procedures, regardless of the type of procedure or where it is performed. Advances in pediatric surgery have occurred as a result of the following [4]:

- Increased recognition of differences between pediatric patients and adults
- More accurate diagnosis and earlier treatment, which has facilitated more favorable outcomes especially in the fetus and preterm neonate
- Greater understanding of the importance of preoperative preparation for the child and parents

DEVELOPMENTAL CONSIDERATIONS

The plan of care should reflect a consideration of the child's age, and interventions should be modified according to the child's developmental stage as identified in Table 1. Developmental theorists emphasize that psychologic growth is the key parameter through which communication is measured. Assessment of psychologic development is based on age-related criteria but includes assessment of individual differences.

Environmental influences on psychologic development include ethnic, cultural, and socioeconomic factors. Erickson [5] presented the most widely used theory of personality development. It is built on Freudian theory but stresses a healthy personality instead of a pathologic approach. Erickson shows specific age-related stages and defines the changes that occur within these stages.

Infant (Birth–1 Year)

The infant experiences two major stressors as a result of hospitalization and the surgical process: separation and pain. Infants' reactions to these stressors include protest (crying), despair, and detachment. Key interventions in caring for the infant are

- Meeting needs promptly
- Allowing unrestricted visiting for parents
- Using comfort measures, such as a pacifier, blanket, special toy, and stroking or patting skin

Toddler (1–3 Years)

The toddler experiences three major stressors in response to surgery and hospitalization: separation, loss of control, and bodily injury and pain. The toddler's loss of control is related to physical restriction, loss of daily routine, and dependency on others. In addition to the reactions experienced by infants, toddlers react with resistance, physical aggression, verbal uncooperativeness, regression, negativism, and temper tantrums. Key interventions in caring for the toddler are

- Allowing them freedom to express feelings of protest within safe limits
- Accepting regressive behavior without commenting
- Incorporating home routine, if possible, and using comfort measures
- Allowing parental visits as soon as possible

Preschool (3–6 Years)

The preschool child experiences the same stressors of separation, loss of control, and bodily injury and pain, but their reactions are much different from those of the toddler. The preschool child's protests are less aggressive and direct. If despair or detachment is shown, it is toward the loss of control. Aggression and regression are the preschooler's reactions to bodily injury and pain. Key interventions for this age group are

- Acknowledging and accepting their fears and anxieties
- Demonstrating equipment with hands-on application
- Encouraging verbalization of feelings
- Allowing parental visits as soon as possible

School-Aged (6–12 Years)

The school-aged child reacts to the same major stressors. However, children in this age group have an increased ability to verbally express feelings, and their reactions to stressors differ greatly. Reactions will vary from isolation and withdrawal, inquisitiveness, and constant, detailed questioning to displaced anger

Table 1
Growth and development

Developmental level	Cognitive Piaget	Psychosocial Erikson	Psychosocial Freud	Moral Kohlberg
Infant (birth to 1 y)	Sensorimotor stage: initial reflex actions become more repetitive and intentional as the infant learns to elicit a response from self or objects in the environment; beginning "object permanence", the ability to understand that an object or person exists even if not seen	Trust vs. mistrust: learns to trust the environment through having basic needs met in an adequate and consistent manner	Oral stage: increases understanding of the environment through activities associated with the mouth (eg, sucking, mouthing, chewing)	Preconventional: determines right and wrong by making decisions according to rules imposed by others or by gratifying impulses; behavior is guided by the expectation of reward or punishment
Toddler (1–3 y)	Sensorimotor stage (until age 2 years): learns cause-and-effect relationships and begins to actively use memory to solve problems; beginning of imitation, speech, and use of symbols; increasing understanding of space and time; advanced concept of object permanence. Preoperational stage (preconceptual, 2–4 years): increasing use of symbols in the form of language and imaginative play; egocentric, unable to view situations from another's perspective	Autonomy vs. shame and doubt: begins to develop independence and control of physical skills and mental processes with the positive encouragement and support of caregivers	Anal stage: develops control over the environment as sphincter control develops	

	Cognitive	Psychosocial	Psychosexual	Moral
Preschool (3–6 y)	Preoperational stage (intuitive, 4–7 years): improves language development, which allows the child to gather information through questioning; less egocentric; unable yet to fully understand the changing or reversible properties of objects	Initiative vs. guilt: initiates goal-directed exploration and manipulation of the self and the environment, with increasing self-confidence and sense of responsibility for actions	Phallic stage: gender identity emerges as a result of unconscious conflict and subsequent identification with the parent of the same sex	Conventional: bases moral behavior on values and expectations of others (eg, family, peers, teachers) and on respect for authority and established rules
School age (6–12 y)	Concrete operational stage (7–11 years): refines logical thought processes by dealing with objects and actions that can be seen and manipulated; develops ability to sort, classify, and order objects, and solve problems systematically and concurrently; understands that certain properties of objects remain the same even though their action or appearance changes (conversation); views a situation from another's perspective	Industry vs. inferiority: develops the ability to achieve and the necessary skills to complete activities and projects successfully, with positive feedback from peers and family	Latency: resolves previous conflicts and develops greater interest in others	Postconventional (autonomous): makes moral, rational decisions based on an understanding of law and social order beyond the immediate environment, and considers right and wrong within the context of what is best for the individual and society as a whole
Adolescence	Formal operational stage (11 years and older): develops abstract reasoning, hypothetical thinking, deduction, and synthesis of information	Identity vs. identity diffusion: develops a positive sense of self, allegiance to a set of values, and mastery of social skills by experimenting with different roles	Genital stage: constructs appropriate relationships with members of the opposite sex	

From Luckman J. Saunders manual of nursing care. Philadelphia: WB Saunders; 1997. p. 472; with permission.

and a display of total frustration. Occasionally, the school-aged child will attempt to show acceptance of procedures and pain by "trying to act brave." Key interventions for school-aged children are

- Allowing expression and acknowledging fears
- Encouraging questions and using more detailed explanations
- Including them in simple decisions about their care
- Increasing hands-on demonstration of equipment

Adolescent (12–18 Years)

The unique world of the teenager can be challenging for health care providers and parents. The adolescent focuses on two stressors: loss of control and bodily injury and pain. The stress of separation, so apparent in the other developmental ages, is experienced when adolescents are separated from their peer group and friends because of prolonged hospitalization and absence from school. The behavioral reactions displayed by teenagers are often as wide and diverse as their mood swings. Key interventions include

- Providing detailed explanations
- Encouraging adjustment to and acceptance of authority figures
- Encouraging questions and allowing expression of feelings
- Respecting privacy
- Including the teenager in decision making and surgical plan of care

Understanding the patient's level of psychologic development can help the caregiver communicate more effectively with the pediatric patient throughout the perioperative experience. Interaction should occur according to individual developmental level regardless of age.

FAMILY-CENTERED CONCEPTS

Facilities that provide pediatric services should have policies on the rights and responsibilities [6] of pediatric patients and their parents or guardians. Many facilities have developed a "bill of rights," such as the one listed in Box 1, that is presented to families at admission and displayed in visible locations.

Legal and ethical considerations, described in Box 2, are also important, especially when caring for pediatric patients. Nurses should be aware of these legal requirements when caring for children.

Informed Consent

Informed consent from the parent or legal guardian of the pediatric patient is required unless the patient is an emancipated minor. An emancipated minor is one who is legally under the age of majority but is recognized as having the legal capacity to consent. Minors may become emancipated through pregnancy, marriage, high school graduation, living independently, and military service. Obtaining assent from patients aged 7 years and older can actively involve the child or adolescent in the decision-making process and is a gesture of respect [5].

Box 1: Bill of rights for children and teens

In this hospital you and your family have the right to:
Respect and personal dignity
Care that supports you and your family
Information you can understand
Quality health care
Emotional support
Care that respects your need to grow, play, and learn
Make choices and decisions

Adapted from Association for the Care of Children's Health: a pediatric bill of rights. Mt. Royal (NJ): Association for the Care of Children's Health; 1998.

Child Abuse and Neglect

Nurses working in the preadmission phase should screen all pediatric patients for abuse and neglect. Child abuse and neglect are defined as "physical or mental injury, sexual abuse or exploitation, negligent treatment or maltreatment" [7]. The perioperative nurse is in a unique position to assess for the presence of abuse because patients are disrobed in the operating room. Each state has a child abuse law [7] that spells out the legal responsibility to report abuse and suspicion of abuse. Nurses are mandated reporters in every state. Failure to report suspected child abuse could result in a fine or other punishment according to individual statutes.

Family Support

Parents remain the greatest source of support for children undergoing surgery. Parenting practices may directly influence the way the patient responds to caregivers and the perioperative environment. Parents cannot be assumed have the knowledge to prepare their children for this experience. Parents need to be given the proper tools and educational resource materials to make informed

---

Box 2: Legal and ethical considerations

The nurse or physician must obtain informed consent before any procedure or treatment that is potentially harmful to the child. These include immunizations and participation in research. A parent, an adolescent older than 18 years, or an emancipated minor (a minor child who is no longer dependent upon parents for either emotional or financial support) may give consent. Children able to understand the procedure and its implications should be included in the decision making. In certain cultures, the primary caregiver is not the child's legal guardian and cannot give consent. To give culturally sensitive care, include all the child's significant caregivers in the decision-making process.

From Luckmann J. Saunders manual of nursing care. Philadelphia: WB Saunders; 1997. p. 475; with permission.

---

decisions that are in the best interest of their child. Numerous articles support the theory that the family experiences less stress when everyone knows and understands what is expected [8].

PREADMISSION TEACHING
Teaching Programs
Preoperative teaching programs for children and their families have been developed to standardize information and reduce perioperative anxiety for the child and parents. Many facilities with large pediatric populations have developed some type of teaching program for the children waiting to undergo surgery and their families. Programs vary greatly and are often influenced by the resources each institution has available.

Teaching is more effective when multiple methodologies, such as those presented in Box 3, are incorporated into the program. However, no single method is effective at every facility or even for every child in the same institution. Appropriate objectives for a teaching program are as follows:

- Identify routines
- Discuss procedures and equipment
- Explain methods used by staff
- Explain medical terminology
- Discuss concerns of child and parents
- Arrange ample question-and-answer time
- Evaluate the program for effectiveness

Children aged 7 to 12 years benefit from preoperative teaching given 1 to 2 weeks before the surgical date, whereas children aged 4 to 7 years benefit from information provided closer to the actual date of surgery [9]. Guidelines that reinforce and review all of the information must be shared with the family as the surgical date approaches.

Box 3: Teaching methodologies

1. Audiovisual: show video of the program; send to families unable to attend
2. Role playing: allow children to dress up in surgical hats, booties, and masks
3. Play therapy: allow children to act out, draw, color, or describe events
4. Handouts: provide children with coloring books depicting events of the surgical day for effective reinforcement tools; information for parents on specific do's and don'ts is particularly helpful as the surgical date approaches
5. Tours: take children on a tour through the operating room, the PACU, and the phase II or discharge area to reduce fear of the unknown
6. Models: allow children to touch and manipulate equipment, as appropriate
7. Question-and-answer time: provide time for parents and children to ask questions; parents also appreciate time to ask questions without children present
8. Evaluation: determine effectiveness of the program

Telephone Screening/Preadmission Testing

Preoperative screening is essential for ensuring compliance with instructions and also discovering any previously unidentified medical conditions [10]. Facilities use preoperative telephone calls or preadmission testing to provide preoperative routines, time schedules, and feeding instructions. The medical history is reviewed and the family is given opportunities to ask questions or report changes in the child's condition. Changes in health status should be reported to the anesthesiologist and surgeon. Individualized instructions can also be given.

PREOPERATIVE PREPARATION

Preoperative requirements for pediatric patients include a complete history and physical; appropriate laboratory tests, if necessary; consultations when indicated; an appropriate fasting period; and a chance for the nurse to personally evaluate and establish a rapport with the child and parents. The data allow the nurse to formulate an effective plan of care for the child [2].

The nursing process is the basis for perioperative care of pediatric patients, and the perioperative assessment is the first phase of the process. Data are gathered and reviewed, nursing diagnoses are formulated, outcomes are identified, and care is planned, implemented, and evaluated. Questions and observations allow the nurse to classify the learning needs of the child and family into one or more of the following learning domains [11]:

Cognitive: needs further knowledge
Affective: needs a change in attitude
Psychomotor: needs to learn a motor skill

Documentation of assessment findings is an important part of the process. All caregivers should have easy access to the communication tool chosen by the facility. Information should be documented in writing, the tool easy to use, and the information recorded in one place. Many facilities have moved to electronic documentation, and the systems should be carefully designed to adequately describe the nursing process.

History and Physical

Physiologic assessment of pediatric patients is compared with national averages when establishing baseline norms. If a child has a systemic disease, it should be under good control. A review of physical systems on the day of surgery allows for discovery of any new symptoms. A baseline set of vital signs is also obtained at this time, including an accurate weight. Further information that should be obtained includes feeding history, medication history, allergies to food or medication, and preclusion of possible latex allergies. Table 2 lists other suggested assessments important for the pediatric patient.

Preoperative Fasting

Families facing surgery or other medical procedures with their infants and young children confront many challenges, such as preoperative fasting. Preoperative fasting attempts to minimize the volume of the gastric fluids left in the

Table 2
Preoperative assessments important to the pediatric patient

Physical	Social	Developmental	Parental
Head circumference	Parental validation of NPO status	Pet names for objects or functions	Understanding of preoperative instructions, especially NPO ramifications
Loose teeth	Preferred name to be called	Use of pacifier, bottle, cup	Availability of child care assistance for travel
Skin: rashes, possible signs of communicable disease	Specific fears	Loved objects	Availability of child car seat/appropriate restraint device
Recent exposure to communicable disease	Typical behavior patterns when in pain	Communication skills and level	Resources for postoperative care of child
Currency of vaccinations		Potty training status	Understanding of potential complications: signs and symptoms, when to call for help
Recent illness of child or siblings			

Data from Ireland D. Pediatric patients and their families. In: Burden N, DeFazio Quinn D, O' Brien D, et al, editors. Ambulatory surgical nursing. 2nd edition. Philadelphia: WB Saunders; 2000. p. 613–42.

stomach and has been believed to reduce the chance of pulmonary aspiration. Clinical research generally supports either 2 or 3 hours of fasting before anesthesia for fully breastfed infants. Some earlier studies have concluded that the rate of gastric emptying for human milk is twice as fast as that for infant formula, but not as fast as for clear liquids [12].

The American Society of Anesthesiologists (ASA) formed a task force in 1996 to review relevant clinical human research studies published from 1966 to 1996. Table 3 shows clinical guidelines for preoperative fasting derived from task force data [13] and approved by the House of Delegates at the 1998 ASA Annual Meeting. Because some facilities have not yet adopted these fasting guidelines, concise and clear instructions must be given to the parents for whichever fasting orders are observed. The importance of following these instructions before undergoing anesthesia must be emphasized.

Preoperative Laboratory Testing

Laboratory requirements vary according to hospital or facility policy. Routine preoperative laboratory testing is no longer recommended [10] in the absence of a definite medical indication. Generally, a hematocrit is ordered for children younger than 1 year [14]. Additional laboratory tests should be ordered on an individual basis, depending on the child's history or the procedure being performed.

Table 3
Preoperative fasting guidelines

Ingested material	Minimum fasting time[a] (h)
Clear liquids[b]	2
Breast milk	4
Infant formula	6
Nonhuman milk	6
Light meal[c]	6

[a]Fasting times apply to all ages.
[b]Water, fruit juice without pulp, carbonated beverages, clear tea, black coffee.
[c]Dry toast and clear liquid.
Data from Development of American Society of Anesthesiologists (ASA) fasting guidelines. Update in Anesthesia: Practical Procedures, Issue 12 (2000) Article 2: page 2 of 2, World Federation of Societies of Anaesthesiologists, world wide web implementation by the NDA Web Team, Oxford.

Preoperative Medication

No one consensus exists on the theory or method of using preanesthesia medication for children. The American Academy of Pediatrics states that drugs should achieve five goals: (1) guard the patient's safety and welfare; (2) minimize physical discomfort or pain; (3) minimize negative psychologic responses to treatment by providing analgesia and maximize the potential for amnesia; (4) control behavior; and (5) return the patient to a state in which safe discharge, as determined by recognized criteria, is possible [15]. However, not all pediatric patients need premedication.

Oral midazolam syrup is used for preoperative sedation of ambulatory patients without prolonging emergence or delaying recovery and discharge times. Sevoflurane has improved the speed and ease of inhalational induction in children. Desflurane is associated with the fastest emergence, but should not be used for induction of anesthesia because of its propensity to cause laryngospasm and coughing. These two agents, however, frequently require an opioid supplement during emergence from anesthesia to reduce the agitation that is frequently associated with a state of rapid alertness [7].

Several drug options are available (Table 4). The medication chosen should be atraumatic, with oral, existing intravenous, rectal, or transmucosal routes preferred. For most children, intramuscular injections cause more anxiety than the surgery and should be avoided unless they are required for specific conditions. The child's response to any form of medication must be carefully monitored. Children should not be allowed to walk around play areas unattended after being medicated. Stretchers should have side rails up and be padded for extra protection. Parents should be instructed on the effects of the medication and how their child's sensorium may change. Normal reactions such as facial flushing and warm skin should be pointed out to avoid alarming the parents. Supplemental oxygen, pulse oximetry, and resuscitation equipment should always be immediately available in the event of respiratory depression, although this rarely occurs at the dosages given to children [3].

Table 4
Medications and dosages commonly used for pediatric premedication

Drug	Route	Usual dose (mg/kg)
Opioids		
Morphine sulfate	Intravenous	0.1–0.3
	Intramuscular	0.1–0.3
	Rectal	Not recommended
Fentanyl	Oral transmucosal	0.015–0.020
	Sublingual	0.010–0.015
	Intravenous	0.001–0.005
Meperidine	Intravenous	1.0–3.0
	Intramuscular	1.0–3.0
	Rectal	Not recommended
Sedatives		
Diazepam	Oral	0.1–0.3
	Intravenous	0.1–0.3
	Intramuscular	Not recommended
	Rectal	0.2–0.3
Midazolam	Oral	0.5–0.75
	Intravenous	0.05–0.15
	Intramuscular	0.05–0.15
	Rectal	0.5–0.75
	Nasal	0.2–0.5
	Sublingual	0.2–0.5
Pentobarbital	Intravenous	1.0–3.0 (maximum 100 mg)
	Intramuscular	5.0–7.0
Chloral hydrate	Orally/rectally	20–75 (maximum 100 mg or 2.0 g)
Ketamine	Oral	3.0–10.0
	Intravenous	1.0–3.0
	Intramuscular	2.0–10.0
	Rectal	5.0–10.0
	Nasal	3.0–5.0
	Sublingual	3.0–5.0
Barbiturates		
Methohexital	Intramuscular	7.0–10.0
	Rectal (10% solution)	20.0–30.0
Thiopental	Intramuscular	7.0–10.0
	Rectal	20.0–30.0
Combinations		
Midazolam	Oral	0.5–0.75
Children's Tylenol		10.0–15.0
Other		
EMLA cream	Topical	Apply ½ of 5-g tube to site. Cover with occlusive transparent dressing
Lidocaine 2.5%	Minor procedure	Apply 60 min
Prilocaine 2.5%	Major procedure	Apply 120–180 min

Data form Wong DL. Whaley & Wong's nursing care of infants and children. 5th edition. St. Louis (MO): Mosby; 1995. p. 1144–5; and Twersky RS. The ambulatory anesthesia handbook. St. Louis (MO): Mosby; 1995. p. 148–51.

PEDIATRIC ANESTHESIA

Preoperative Assessment by the Anesthesia Provider

A preoperative visit by the anesthesia provider is a vital part of preparation for the pediatric patient. During physical assessment [3] special attention is given to the heart, lungs, and upper airways. Loose teeth are noted. An ASA physical status classification is assigned to the pediatric patient.

Types of Induction

Depending on institutional policy, parents may be present during induction to comfort the child and reduce separation anxiety. Before entering the operating room, parents should be well informed as to what they may see or hear and how their child may react. The perioperative nurse should also make parents aware that they may be asked to leave the room if an emergency arises [16].

Distraction techniques for mask anesthesia are useful tools used by the perioperative nurse to minimize a child's stress and anxiety. Story telling, singing softly, or blowing bubbles are effective distraction techniques (Fig. 1). Types of induction include [3]

- Inhaled
- Rectal
- Intravenous infusion
- Ketamine

ANESTHESIA CONSIDERATIONS

Anesthesia is approached differently in pediatric patients compared with adults. Equipment and supplies for the pediatric airway (Table 5) are scaled down and different anesthesia circuits and delivery systems are often used. Face mask, laryngeal mask airway, and endotracheal tube are the most common techniques used to administer general anesthesia to pediatric patients [16].

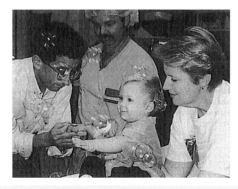

Fig. 1. The use of distraction technique during induction. (*From* Maldonado SS, LeBoeuf MB. Pediatric surgery. In: Rothrock JC, editor. Alexander's care of the patient in surgery. 12th edition. Philadelphia: Mosby; 2003. p. 1218; with permission.)

Table 5
Sizes for pediatric airway equipment

Age	Laryngoscope	Endotracheal tube size	Suction catheter (French)
Infant (birth–12 mo)	Miller 0–1	2.5–4.5 (uncuffed)	5–8
Toddler (1–3 y)	Miller 2 Flagg 2	4.5 (uncuffed)	8
Preschool-age child (4–5 y)	Miller 2 Flagg 2	5.0 (uncuffed)	10
School-age child (6–12 y)	Miller 2 MacIntosh 2	5.5–7.0 (uncuffed to age of 8 y)	10–12
Adolescent (13–20 y)	MacIntosh 3 Miller 3	7.0–8.0 (cuffed)	12

Data from Maldonado SS, LeBoeuf MB. Pediatric surgery. In: Rothrock JC, editor. Alexander's care of the patient in surgery, 12th edition. Philadelphia: Mosby; 2003. p. 1211–93.

ANATOMIC AND PHYSIOLOGIC DIFFERENCES
Pediatric Airway

Compared with adults, children have definite anatomic and physiologic differences, some of which are shown in Fig. 2. The infant's head is proportionately larger in comparison with the body. The infant and child's nares are narrow, and the tongue is large. Infants are obligate nasal breathers. The larynx is high and funnel shaped, causing a natural narrowing at the cricoid ring. This rigid

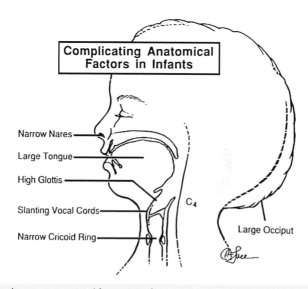

Complicating Anatomical Factors in Infants

Narrow Nares
Large Tongue
High Glottis
Slanting Vocal Cords
Narrow Cricoid Ring
Large Occiput
C₄

Fig. 2. Complicating anatomical factors in infants. (*From* Barash PG, Cullen BF, Stoelting RK. Handbook of clinical anesthesia. 3rd edition. Philadelphia: Lippincott-Raven; 1997. p. 390; with permission.)

circular framework of cartilage contains the epiglottis and glottis (vocal cords). The epiglottis is very high, almost to the soft palate, and is omega shaped and protrudes over the larynx about 45°. Vocal cords are slanted, and in infancy the glottis is located more cephalad than in later childhood. Laryngeal reflexes are very active. The tracheal diameter is small and is located downward and posterior; this diameter triples in size by 12 years of age.

Respiratory System

The chest wall is very compliant and the ribs are more horizontal; therefore the infant is mechanically disadvantaged. The muscles are still immature and fatigue easily. Breathing is predominantly diaphragmatic in the neonate. The respiratory center is immature and is easily depressed by the effects of sedatives, anesthetic agents, and opioids.

Cardiovascular System

The myocardium of the neonate is immature and less compliant. In attempting to meet oxygen requirements, the cardiac output of the infant is 30% to 50% greater than that of adults. The neonate has a high vagal tone manifested by bradycardia. Blood pressure readings vary more frequently in infants because of sleep and activity patterns. Systolic and diastolic readings continue to increase from the newborn period until the child reaches adolescence, when pressure readings assume adult levels. Table 6 provides an example of normal vital signs. Hypotension in an infant is not apparent until 50% of the circulating volume is lost, and is usually caused by myocardial depression from anesthetic agents, primarily inhalation anesthesia.

Renal System

Preterm renal function is abnormal because of tubular immaturity. The creatinine clearance at 28 weeks is only 25% of a full-term neonate [17]. By the

Table 6
Normal vital signs by age

Age	Degrees Fahrenheit	Degrees Celsius	Pulse rate (beats/min)	Respiratory rate (breaths/min)	Blood pressure (mm Hg)
Newborn	96.8–99 axillary	36–37.2 axillary	120–160	30–60	Systolic: 46–92 Diastolic: 38–71
3 y	97.5–98.6 axillary	36.4–37 axillary	80–125	20–30	Systolic: 72–110 Diastolic: 40–73
10 y	97.5–98.6 oral	36.4–37 oral	70–110	16–22	Systolic: 83–121 Diastolic: 45–79
16 y	97.5–98.6 oral	36.4–37 oral	55–90	15–20	Systolic: 93–131 Diastolic: 49–85

Temperature readings will vary depending on the method used.
   After the age 12 years, a boy's pulse rate is 5 beats/min slower than a girl's.
   After the age 14 years, a boy's blood pressure is higher than in a girl's.
   Data from James SR, Ashwill JW, Droske SC. Nursing care of children. 2nd edition. Philadelphia: WB Saunders; 2002. p. 235.

age of 1 year, the glomerular filtration rate (GFR) is equivalent to that of an adult. Because of tubular immaturity, the premature neonate is less able to reabsorb glucose and bicarbonate, leading to metabolic acidosis and dehydration.

Thermoregulation

Neonates are less able to maintain their body temperature. They have a very large surface area–to–volume ratio, little subcutaneous fat, and also a large head. Infants can lose up to 75% of their body heat through head exposure to room air. Infants younger than 3 months do not have a shiver response. Body temperature in the newborn ranges from as low as 97°F to 100°F (36.1°C–37.7°C).

A hypothermic newborn or infant metabolizes anesthetic agents more slowly and is susceptible to postoperative respiratory depression and delayed emergence from anesthesia. The first sign of hypothermia in a child younger than 1 year is a heart rate less than 100 beats per minute [3]. Oxygen consumption is at a minimum when abdominal skin temperature is 97°F (36.1°C). A room temperature 5°F (−15°C) cooler than that of abdominal skin produces a 50% increase in oxygen consumption, creating the risk for acidosis. Neonates, infants, and children are kept warm during surgery to minimize heat loss and prevent hypothermia. Wrapping the head and exposed extremities helps prevent this heat loss.

Hyperthermia during surgery can be the result of several factors, including

- Dehydration
- Decreased sweating from atropine administration
- Fever
- Excessive drapes
- Drugs, such as barbiturates and anesthetic agents, that disturb temperature regulation

Distribution and Metabolism

The blood–brain barrier is poorly developed in the infant, and therefore the entry of drugs such as narcotics is increased by 20% to 100%. The liver is the most immature of all the gastrointestinal organs during infancy and remains functionally immature until after the first year of life. Because many drugs are released hepatically, this immaturity increases the half-life of many agents.

COMMON PEDIATRIC SURGICAL PROCEDURES

Pediatric surgery encompasses all specialties but can generally be divided into three major areas: congenital malformations or defects; acquired diseases of infancy and childhood; and trauma. The pediatric patient adapts well to various surgical procedures (Table 7), many of which can be performed in an outpatient setting.

POSTANESTHESIA CARE AND CONCERNS

Postanesthesia Care Unit: Phase I

Children should be transferred from the operating room to the PACU by the anesthesia team and the operating room nurse. The anesthesia caregiver should give a full report to the PACU nurse. Initial monitoring in the PACU includes respiratory rate, blood pressure, pulse oximetry, EKG, fluid balance, and temperature control. When vital signs are obtained (see Table 6), the PACU values should be compared with the preoperative and intraoperative recordings. The pulse oximeter is superior to clinical judgment in providing the earliest warning of a desaturation event [18]. Vital signs should be assessed every 15 minutes (or more frequently if the condition or extent of the surgery warrants) for the duration of the initial postoperative period. The child should be positioned according to the procedure performed. Prone and semiprone positions facilitate drainage and help prevent aspiration if the child vomits.

A patent intravenous line should be maintained in the postoperative care unit. In ambulatory surgery, additional intravenous fluids may not be necessary if the intraoperative total fluid volume is sufficient to cover the initial postoperative recovery. However, a patent intravenous line should be maintained throughout recovery. In the event of postoperative vomiting, additional fluids may be necessary.

All children who have been given anesthesia are classified as a 1:1 nurse–patient acuity until reflexes and consciousness return. Nurse–patient ratios are addressed in Resource 3 of the *Standards of Perianesthesia Nursing* published by the American Society of Perianesthesia Nurses (ASPAN) [19]. Safety devices such as side rails, bumper pads, seat belts, stretcher safety straps, and arm restraints should be used as needed to protect children from injury.

Individual policies vary, but many facilities now allow parents to join their children in the phase I PACU [20]. Length of stay is generally established by the anesthesia department. Pediatric patients should not be released from phase I until they are awake, have returned to their baseline preoperative status, and meet specific discharge criteria developed by the anesthesia department.

The anesthesiologist is responsible for determining preoperative and postoperative fluid deficits. Fluid replacement is determined by various factors: (1) number of hours the child was NPO before surgery; (2) hours of surgery; and (3) blood loss. Proper fluid balance must be corrected and maintained because energy is used in maintaining ventilation, cardiac output, regulating temperature, and muscle activity.

COMPLICATIONS AND TREATMENT

In general, the major complications seen in the postanesthesia care unit are respiratory problems. The rate and depth of ventilation should be monitored in the PACU. Respiratory depression occurs with greater frequency if muscle relaxants are used during anesthesia. The most common respiratory complications include

- Airway obstruction
- Secretions/suctioning

Table 7
Common pediatric surgical procedures

Surgery	Definition	Indications for surgery	Nursing considerations	Discharge instructions
Strabismus repair	Surgery to correct misalignment of one or both eyes	Unresponsive to medical regimen of patching; avoid permanent impairment of vision; improve cosmetic appearance	Restrain if necessary to avoid pulling at eyes and dressings Provide comfort by medicating for pain/nausea. Decrease stimulation and dim lights Reunite with parents as soon as possible	Stress importance of not rubbing eyes Observe for signs of infection: redness, matting, and discolored drainage Reassure parents that tears may be blood-tinged initially Decrease stimulation and light Call physician if eyes become malaligned or signs of infection occur
Myringotomy with/without tympanostomy tubes	Facilitate drainage of fluid and allow continued ventilation of middle ear	Treatment for chronic otitis media	Provide comfort by medicating for pain Pulling/tugging may indicate pain Observe color and amount of drainage	Keep water out of ears during bath/shower Earplugs may be recommended Swimming, diving, jumping, and submerging are usually discouraged Parents should be instructed that tube may fall out naturally
Adenoidectomy	Removal of the adenoids	Recurrent otitis media, hearing loss, nasal airway obstruction: heavy snoring, heavy respirations, and nasal speech	Observe for signs of increased bleeding: increased bleeding from nose, tachycardia, pallor, frequent clearing of throat, restlessness, vomiting bright red blood Position for drainage Medicate for pain Encourage fluids when reactive and bleeding and emesis is under control	Avoid irritating tender tissue Give soft foods that are cool and bland Use analgesics as ordered Observe for signs of infection: increased temperature, severe earache, and cough Quiet household activities, increase per physician's instructions Instruct parents that tonsil scab falls off 5–10 days postoperatively

Tonsillectomy	Removal of palatine tonsils	Massive hypertrophy, obstruction of airway, difficulty eating, malignancy, and chronic tonsillitis	Same as above	Same as above
Herniorrhaphy	Prolapse of a portion of the intestine into the inguinal ring; most common infant procedure	Persistent painless inguinal swelling, partial obstruction of bowel, and incarcerated hernia	Comfort measures: pain medication or injection of local at site Position with pillows under knees Change diapers often	Observe for signs of infection: redness, tenderness, increased temperature Frequent diaper changes Sponge baths first 2–5 days Older children should be cautioned against lifting, pushing, wrestling, and athletics for 2–3 week
Hydrocelectomy	Presence of fluid in the persistent processus vaginalis	Communicating hydrocele that does not resolve in 1 year; potential for herniation	Same as with hernia Advise parents that temporary swelling and discoloration of scrotum resolves spontaneously	Same as above
Hypospadias	Urethral opening is located below the glans pens or anywhere along the ventral surface of the penile shaft	Enable child to void in standing position with voluntary direction of urine in normal manner; improved physical appearance for psychologic reasons produce sexually adequate organ	Prepare parents and child for type of procedure and what results to expect Urinary diversion sometimes necessary for optimum healing May have indwelling catheter or stent. Restrain as necessary Medicate for pain	Teach parents catheter care: avoid kinking, twisting, or blocking catheter/stent Show how to empty urine bag Encourage fluid intake, bathing twice daily, wearing loose clothing, and avoidance of sandboxes, straddle-type toys, swimming, and rough activity until physician permits

(continued on next page)

Table 7
(continued)

Surgery	Definition	Indications for surgery	Nursing considerations	Discharge instructions
Orchiopexy	Undescended testes brought down into the scrotum and secured in position	If undescended spontaneously Surgery performed between age 1–2 years to prevent damage to testicle by exposure to higher body heat, tumor formation, trauma and torsion, cosmetic and psychologic handicap	Comfort measures: medicate for pain/ nausea Position with pillows under knees Injection with local at sire is helpful Usually performed as outpatient	Instruct parents on prevention of infection: show proper cleaning of site Frequent cleaning after urination and bowel movements Restrict activity Provide counseling referral to family for questions on fertility
Closed reduction of fracture	Bone fragments realigned and immobilize by traction or by closed manipulation and casting	To regain alignment and length of bony fragments (reduction); to retain alignment and length (immobilization); to restore function to injured parts	Observe neurovascular status; check regularly for edema, allow cast to dry uncovered Medicate for pain	Instruct parents on cast care and proper positioning Show how to check for adequate circulation Avoid small items that can be put inside cast by small children
Cleft lip repair	Deficiency of tissue (skin, muscle, and mucosa) along one or both sides of the upper lip or, rarely, in the midline results in a cleft at the site of deficiency	To approximate the normal lip as closely as possible Early surgical correction aids in feeding and infant–parent bonding	Timing of repair follows the "rule of 10": the infant is 10 weeks of age, weighs 10 lb, and has hemoglobin of 10 Usually around 3 months of age.	Logan bow dressing applied to the cheeks with tape strips, and elbow restraints are applied to inhibit pulling, touching Instruct on good oral care and follow diet instructions

Cleft palate	A separation or cleft of the palate occurs in the midline and may involve only the soft palate or both the hard and soft palates	To aid in the production of normal speech sounds An intact hard palate is necessary to prevent escape of air through the nose during speech and to prevent the egress of liquid and food from the nose	A pharyngeal flap may be part of the primary cleft palate repair to reduce the size of the opening between the oropharynx and nasopharynx, thus eliminating the nasal escape of air during speech and decreasing the hypernasality or "cleft palate speech"	Instruct on oral care, diet instructions Speech therapy may be indicated
Pectus excavatum	Congenital malformation of the chest wall, characterized by a pronounced funnel-shaped, concave depression over the lower end of the sternum	To reduce cardiopulmonary impairment in severe cases and also decrease exercise intolerance and chest pain in the moderate to severe forms	Minimally invasive procedure where curved metal bar is slid under the ribs to elevate sunken portion No ribs or cartilage is removed Bar is individually tailored to recipient Must be removed 1–2 years later and removal can be performed as outpatient	Less complicated in younger children because cartilage is softer and less calcified Teens and young adults can have the procedure performed successfully but osseous tissue is less flexible
Ventriculoatrial and ventriculoperitoneal shunts	Hydrocephalus may be congenital or acquired Associated with blockage in the ventricular drainage system	Prevent cranial distortion caused by the increasing size of the ventricles	Air trapping in the valve assembly should be avoided Unit must be handled with extreme care Follow specific manufacturer's instructions for implantable devices	Keep free of lint, powder, or other foreign bodies Instruct on care to prevent obstruction, disconnection, and malfunction and educate on signs of infection

Data from Wong DL. Whaley & Wong's nursing care of infants and children. 5th edition. St. Louis (MO): CV Mosby; 1995; Luckman J. Sanders manual of nursing care. Philadelphia: WB Saunders; 1997; Maldonado SS, LeBoeuf MB. Pediatric surgery. In: Rohrock JC. Alexander's care of the patient in surgery. 12th edition. St. Louis (MO): Mosby; 2003; and Litwack K. Core curriculum for post anesthesia nursing practice. 3rd edition. Philadelphia: WB Saunders; 1995.

- Stridor
- Postintubation croup
- Laryngeal edema/obstruction
- Laryngospasm
- Respiratory depression
- Bronchospasm

Nonrespiratory complications seen in the PACU include nausea and vomiting, aspiration, emergence delirium, and malignant hyperthermia (MH). Although not considered a specific complication, postoperative pain can significantly enhance any of the respiratory complications and should be managed appropriately.

Airway Obstruction

Every pediatric patient, particularly children who have been intubated during anesthesia, should be monitored for signs of airway obstruction. Although infants are obligatory nasal breathers, the large tongue tends to fall back and produce pharyngeal obstruction and may also adhere to the roof of the mouth. Manipulations such as pulling the chin forward, using a pacifier, and holding the infant in a sitting position may be successful in loosening the tongue. Hyperextension of the jaws in the infant results in obstruction rather than clearing.

Secretions/Suctioning

Excessive secretions can rapidly obstruct the airway and cause respiratory problems. Properly positioning the child to facilitate drainage can eliminate many risks associated with secretions. When positioning is not effective, suctioning must be performed carefully with a proper size suction catheter (see Table 5). The infant's nares should be suctioned first because of the obligate nasal breathing. Excessive or overly deep suctioning may trigger a laryngospasm.

Stridor/Postintubation Croup

The "crowing" sound of stridor is unmistakable and is most often seen in children who have been intubated during surgery. Postintubation croup is caused by glottic or tracheal edema. When laryngeal edema occurs, the diameter of an infant or small child's airway can become significantly reduced; 1 mm of edema in the infant's trachea at the cricoid level decreases the diameter of the airway by 75% [21].

Postintubation croup is a frequent complication after traumatic intubation, prolonged intubation, improper endotracheal tube size, excessive coughing on the endotracheal tube, and surgical trauma. An increased incidence occurs in the 1- to 4-year-old age group. Postintubation croup is often accompanied by stridor and is characterized by a "barklike" cough. Treatment for stridor and postintubation croup is similar:

- Calm reassurance
- Oxygen mist, which may be recommended overnight, depending on severity; if a tent is used, it can be referred to as "raindrops" or a "rain forest" to reduce fear

- Nebulized racemic epinephrine (0.5 mL of a 2.25% solution in 2.5 mL of normal saline)
- Corticosteroids, such as dexamethasone (dexamethasone, 0.2 mg/kg, intravenously), to decrease laryngeal inflammation, although these remain controversial [22]
- Reintubation if condition is severe or worsens after initial treatment

Racemic epinephrine is used for its vasoconstrictive properties and has a well-known rebound phenomena. Within 2 hours, the clinical effects dissipate and the edema and obstruction can be worse than before. The child should be closely monitored [23,24] to detect any signs of possible rebound.

Laryngeal Edema/Obstruction

Irritation from the endotracheal tube and suctioning can cause edema. The most common cause of laryngeal edema/obstruction is the use of inappropriate-sized endotracheal tubes for intubation. Cuffed endotracheal tubes are never used in children younger than 7 to 8 years because they reduce the lumen size, increase airway resistance, and place pressure on the tracheal mucosa. The symptoms of laryngeal obstruction, in order of appearance, are croupy cough, hoarseness, inspiratory stridor, and aphonia (no sound). Early signs of impending airway obstruction include increased pulse and respiratory rate; substernal, suprasternal, and intercostal retractions; flaring nares; and increased restlessness [5]. Treatment includes high, humidified oxygen therapy; body hydration; antibiotics (if infection is a contributing factor); and corticosteroids.

Laryngospasm

Laryngospasm may occur on emergence from anesthesia. Children who have irritable airways are especially prone to this complication. *Laryngospasm* is airway obstruction that occurs when the muscles of the larynx force the vocal cords to close because of blood or secretions on the vocal cords, inhalation of irritant gases, irritation from the endotracheal tube or oral airway, or too excessive suctioning. Characteristics, in order of appearance, are dyspnea, "crowing" sound on inspiration, rocking motion of chest wall indicating accessory muscle use, and aphonia. Aphonia indicates that a total blockage has occurred. Treatment of laryngospasm requires the following:

- Remaining calm and assembling additional help during early warning signs
- Administering 100% oxygen and positive-pressure ventilation while maintaining end-expiratory pressure to open the cords
- Oropharyngeal suctioning to possibly remove secretions that precipitated the spasm
- Administering succinylcholine if spasm is unrelieved by positive-pressure
- Airway and ventilation support if muscle relaxants are required; possible reintubation

Continued observation and monitoring after the spasm has resolved are absolutely necessary. Postobstructive pulmonary edema, also called *noncardiogenic pulmonary edema*, may develop after laryngospasm, especially in children [24,25].

Respiratory Depression

Respiratory depression is seen in children for various reasons. The most common causes are inadequate reversal of muscle relaxants causing a residual neuromuscular blockade; residual effects of inhalation agents, barbiturates, and narcotics; and a preexisting pulmonary disease. Treatment can include any or all of the following: a "stir-up regimen" of verbal and tactile stimulation, reversal agents to reverse narcotic-induced depression, reversal agents to reverse the effects of nondepolarizing relaxants, and, at a minimum, close, continuous monitoring of oxygen saturation and respiratory effort.

Bronchospasm

Bronchospasm is another complication that results in diminished ventilation. It is more common in children who have a preexisting bronchospastic disease, such as asthma. High-pitched wheezing is an indication of this spasm and can be heard on auscultation along with coarse rails. In addition to positioning and oxygen therapy, parenteral and inhaled bronchodilating drugs, such as intravenous aminophylline and isoetharine and metaproterenol inhalers, may be used to treat this condition.

Aspiration

Aspiration of gastric secretions produces complications in pediatric patients that are similar to those experienced by adults. The aspirated secretions may cause irritation to the trachea and bronchi. The diagnosis is made on the basis of tachypnea, dyspnea, bronchospasm, cyanosis, shock, and pulmonary edema. Treatment includes positioning the child's head down and turned to one side to facilitate drainage; suctioning; administering oxygen through face mask; confirming aspiration through diagnostic; and supporting respiratory and cardiovascular systems.

Emergence Delirium

Some patients emerge from general anesthesia in a state of "excitement," characterized by restlessness, disorientation, crying, moaning, irrational talking, and inappropriate behavior. The incidence of emergence delirium is higher among children. It is a completely dissociative state and the child is amnesic during the entire episode, which can last from 30 seconds to 5 minutes. Medications, pain, and a full bladder are believed to be leading causes, and protecting the child from injury is the nurse's primary responsibility during these episodes. Children will fall back to sleep (normally or through the administration of medication) and reawaken calmly without recollection of the incident.

Malignant Hyperthermia

MH is a genetically determined condition triggered by certain general inhalation anesthetics, depolarizing skeletal muscle relaxants, amide local anesthetics, and stress. Research has helped reduce the morbidity and mortality of this syndrome. The incidence of MH ranges from 1 in 14,000 to 15,000 children. The onset of MH usually occurs during induction of anesthesia. Once the acute episode is treated in the operating room, the patient is admitted to the PACU. Recurrence of MH in the PACU has been reported and successful management depends on early assessment and prompt intervention [21].

The presenting symptoms are likely to be end-tidal carbon dioxide levels or rigidity of the jaw (masseter muscle rigidity). This rigidity sometimes does not occur, and the anesthesiologist is then presented with an unexplained tachycardia. Other signs that occur are dark blood in the operative field, ventricular arrhythmias, skin color changes, skeletal muscle rigidity, and, very late in the crisis, the high temperatures for which the condition is named. The anesthesiologist/surgical team must respond immediately to the early signs exhibited, stop all anesthesia, hyperventilate with 100% oxygen, and terminate surgery as quickly as possible. Dantrolene sodium is the only pharmacologic agent known to be effective in the treatment of MH, and its administration should begin immediately. Recommended dosage is 2 to 3 mg/kg as an initial bolus repeated every 5 to 10 minutes until symptoms are controlled. Occasionally a total dose of 10 mg/kg or more may be required [26]. Dantrolene is mixed with sterile water and should be preservative free because of the large amounts that are used. Recognition and treatment of arrhythmias along with correction of the associated acidosis and electrolyte imbalance should be anticipated. The most successful outcome occurs when the syndrome is identified and treated early [27].

The routine use of succinylcholine is contraindicated in children and should only be used for emergency tracheal intubation or when immediate securing of the airway is necessary. Children and adolescents who have undiagnosed myopathies who are administered succinylcholine can experience acute, fulminating destruction of skeletal muscle (rhabdomyolysis) that results in hyperkalemia and cardiac arrest [21].

POSTOPERATIVE PAIN MANAGEMENT

Children deserve and should receive adequate pain management. Until recently, common fallacies about pain in the pediatric population claimed that infants do not feel pain, children have better pain tolerance than adults have, children cannot tell the health care provider where they hurt, children always tell the truth about pain, children become accustomed to pain or painful procedures, behavioral manifestations reflect pain intensity, and narcotics are more dangerous for children than they are for adults [16].

The aim in postoperative pain management is to have children be cooperative, recover quickly, and have minimal side effects. Research into pediatric pain management has shown that infants do demonstrate behavioral and physiologic indicators of pain. Children are able to indicate pain, and children as old as 3 years of age can use pain-rating scales [16]. Assessment methods (pain rating scales or tools) provide a subjective measurement of pain. Many pain scales exist (see Box 4) and should be selected based on the child's age, abilities, and preference.

Box 4
Resource 3
Patient Classification/Recommened Staffing Guidelines

Staffing Is Based on Patient Acuity, Census, And Physical Facility. The Professional Perianesthesia Nurse Uses Prudent Judgment In Determining Nurse: Patient Ratios And Staffing Mix To Reflect Patient Acuity And Nursing Intensity.

PREANESTHESIA PHASE

Preadmission

The professional perianesthesia nursing roles during this phase focus on assessing the patient and developing a plan of care designed to meet the preprocedural physical, psychological, educational, sociocultural, and spiritual needs of the patient/family/significant other. The nursing roles also focus on preparing the patient/family/significant other for his or her experience throughout the perianesthesia continuum. Interviewing and assessment techniques are used to identify potential or actual problems that may occur.

Day of Surgery/Procedure

The professional perianesthesia nursing roles during this phase focus on validation of existing information and completion of preparation of the patient for his or her experience. The professional registered nurse continues to assess the patient and develops a plan of care designed to meet the physical, psychological, educational, sociocultural, and spiritual needs of the patient/family/significant other.

Staffing in the Preanesthesia Phase

Staffing shall be based on, but not limited to, the following criteria:

1. Number of patients.

2. Number of operating rooms.

3. Average time in patient preparation (i.e., education, testing, medication administration).

4. Patient acuity and intensity of care.

5. Procedures (i.e., insertion of invasive lines, regional blocks).

POSTANESTHESIA PHASE

Phase I Level of Care

The professional perianesthesia nursing roles during this phase focus on providing postanesthesia nursing care to the patient in the immediate postanesthesia period, and transitioning them to Phase II level of care, the inpatient setting, or to an intensive care setting for continued care.

CLASS 1:2 ONE NURSE TO TWO PATIENTS WHO ARE

a. one unconscious, stable, without artificial airway, and over the age of 8 years; and one conscious, stable and free of complications.

b. two conscious, stable, and free of complications.

c. two conscious, stable, 8 years of age and under, with family or competent support staff present.

CLASS 1:1 ONE NURSE TO ONE PATIENT

a. at the time of admission, until the critical elements are met.

b. requiring mechanical life support and/or artificial airway.

c. any unconscious patient 8 years of age and under.

d. a second nurse must be available to assist as necessary.

CLASS 2:1 TWO NURSE TO ONE PATIENT

a. one critically ill, unstable, complicated patient.

Two Licensed Nurses, One Of Whom Is A RN Competent In Phase I Post Anesthesia Nursing, Are Present* Whenever A Patient Is Receiving Phase I Level Of Care.

Phase II Level of Care

The professional perianesthesia nursing roles during this phase focus on preparing the patient/family/significant other for care in the home, Phase III level of care or the extended care environment.

CLASS 1:3 ONE NURSE TO THREE PATIENTS

a. Over 8 years of age.

b. 8 years of age and under with family present.

CLASS 1:2 ONE NURSE TO TWO PATIENTS

a. 8 years of age and under without family or support staff present.

b. initial admission of patient procedure.

CLASS 1:1 ONE NURSE TO ONE PATIENT

a. unstable patient of any age requiring transfer.

Two Competent Personnel, One Of Whom Is A RN Competent In Phase II Postanesthesia Nursing, Are Present* Whenever A Patient Is Receiving Phase II Level Of Care. A RN Must Be Present* At All Times During Phase II.

Phase III Level of Care

The professional perianesthesia nursing roles in this phase focus on providing the ongoing care for those patients requiring extended observation/intervention after transfer/discharge from Phase I and Phase II levels of care. Interventions are directed toward preparing the patient/family/significant other for self-care or care by family/significant other.

CLASS 1:3/5 ONE NURSE TO THREE-FIVE PATIENTS

Phase III staffing is dictated by patient acuity and intensity of nursing care. Care is managed by the RN competent in the Phase III level of care. The nurse:patient ratio is not to exceed one nurse to five patients.

Examples of patients that may be cared for in this phase include but are not limited to:

1. Patients awaiting transportation home.

2. Patients with no care giver.
3. Patients who have had procedures requiring extended observation/interventions (i.e., potential risk for bleeding, pain management, PONV, etc.).

ASPAN defines "present" as being in the particular place where the patients is receiving care.

Reference
American Heart Association. PALS Provider Manual. ISBN 0-87493-322-6, 2002.
California Nurses Association sponsored Safe Staffing Law, AB 394. Available at: http://www.leginfo.ca.gov/pub/99-00/bill/asm/ab_0351-0400/ab_394_bill_19991010_chaptered.pdf. Last accessed 12/30/03.

Copyright 2004 American Society of PeriAnesthesia Nurses.

One of the oldest and most extensively tested tools is the Oucher pain scale. The Oucher, originally developed by Beyer in 1980, is a color, laminated poster instrument designed for children as young as 3 years of age [28]. Although most of the validity testing has been completed on children as old as 12 years, the Oucher has also been used successfully on adolescents [29–31]. A recent study determining the adequacy of the alternate forms reliability of three versions of the Oucher pain scale [31]–Caucasian, African-American, and Hispanic–showed that scores for the small and large posters were strong, positive, and significant for all three versions in 3- to 12-year-old children. These results provided evidence of the adequacy of the alternate forms reliability of these scales.

Parental involvement in pain management is vital. Parents know their child's normal behavior and can provide insight into behaviors exhibited in the perioperative setting [14,32]. Effective pain management requires a willingness to use various methods and modalities to achieve optimal results (Table 8). Pharmacologic methods include the administration of narcotic and nonnarcotic analgesics (Table 9). Patient-controlled analgesia is an option for children, as studies have shown that children can successfully use this modality with appropriate instruction and support. Nonpharmacologic methods include distraction, relaxation, guided imagery, and behavioral contracting. Nonpharmacologic methods should never be used as a substitute for appropriate medication but instead should be used to enhance the management of pain [16].

Regardless of the pain intervention used, the results must be evaluated. Careful monitoring and assessment/reassessment are necessary to document the effectiveness of pain management. Research continues, and ignoring the pain children experience will soon be unacceptable, socially and medically [32,33].

PHASE II DISCHARGE CRITERIA AND INSTRUCTIONS

The child must return to baseline level of functioning. Individual facilities have predetermined criteria that must be met before the child is discharged home or

Table 8
Age-specific pain measurement tools for children

Name	Features	Age range	Advantages	Limitations
Visual analog scale	Horizontal 10-cm ruler; subject marks between "no pain" and "worst pain imaginable"	≥8 years	Good psychometric properties: gold standard	Cannot be used in younger children or children who have cognitive limitations
Faces scales (eg, Wong Baker, Oucher, Bieri, McGrath)	Subjects compare their pain to line drawings of faces or photos of children	≥4 years	More useful for younger ages than visual analog scale	Choice of anchors affects responses (neutral versus smiling)
Behavioral or combined behavioral-physiologic scales (eg, CHEOPS, OPS, FACS, NIPS)	Scoring of observed behaviors (eg, facial expression, limb movement) ± heart rate and blood pressure	Some work for any age; others are age-specific	Can be used even for infants and nonverbal children	Overrates fear in toddlers and preschool children Underrates persistent pain Some inconvenient measures requiring videotaping and complex processing
Autonomic measures (eg, heart rate, blood pressure, heart rate spectral analyses)	Scores changes in heart rate, blood pressure, or measures of heart rate variability (eg, "vagal tone")	All ages	All ages Useful for mechanically ventilated patients	Nonspecific; changes can occur unrelated to pain
Color analog scales	Horizontal or vertical ruler, on which increasing intensity of red signifies more pain	≥ 4 years	Useful for younger ages Converges to visual analog scale at older ages	Cannot be used in toddlers or children who have cognitive limitations
Hormonal-metabolic measures	Plasma or salivary sampling of hormones (eg, cortisol, epinephrine)	All ages	Can be used at all ages	Nonspecific; changes can occur unrelated to pain Inconvenient; cannot provide real-time information

Data from Behrman R, Kliegman R, Jenson H. Nelson's textbook of pediatrics. 16th edition. Philadelphia: WB Saunders; 2000. p. 307.

Table 9
Commonly used analgesic drugs and dosages

Drug (trade name)	Dose mg/kg	Route	Duration	Comments/Maximum dose (mg/kg/d)
Nonopioid				
Acetaminophen (eg, Tylenol)	10–15	Oral	Every 4 h	60–90
	30–40	Rectal (1st dose then 20)		Unknown
				Most widely used in children
Aspirin	10–15	Oral	Every 4 h	60
Ibuprofen (Motrin)	5–10	Oral	Every 6–8 h	40
				Used commonly with children
Ketorolac (Toradol)	0.5	IV, IM Oral	Every 6 h	2
	Adolescents: 10 mg/dose		Every 6–8 h	40 mg/d short-term use only; should not be used for more than 5 d
Opioids				
Morphine	0.05–0.1	IV, IM	2–4 h	Seizures in newborns; also in all patients at high doses; avoid in asthmatics and in circulatory compromise MS Contin 8–12-h duration
Meperidine	0.5–1	IV, IM	2–4 h	Catastrophic interactions with MAOIs; metabolite produces seizures; not recommended for long-term use
Fentanyl	0.001	IV	0.5–1 h	Bradycardia; minimal hemodynamic alterations Chest wall rigidity (>5 µg/kg rapid IV bolus). Prescribe naloxone or paralyze with succinylcholine or pancuronium. 80–100 times more potent than morphine.

Codeine	0.5–1	Oral	4–6 h	Oral only Prescribe with acetaminophen
Hydromorphone (Dilaudid)	0.015–0.02	IV	3–4 h	Less CNS depression than morphine; less itching, nausea than morphine; can also be used in IV and epidural PCA 5–7 times more potent than morphine
Oxycodone (Roxicodone)	0.05–0.15	Oral	4–6 h	AHCPR dosage guideline is 0.2 mg/kg Percocet, Tylox, Roxicet

Abbreviations: AHCPR, Agency of Health Care Policy and Research; IM, intramuscularly; IV, intravenously; MAOI, monoamine oxidase inhibitor; PCA; patient-controlled analgesia.

Data from DiMaggio T. Pediatric pain management. In: St. Marie B, editor. Core curriculum for pain management nursing. Philadelphia: WB Saunders; 2002. p. 374–9; and Ireland D. Pediatric patients and their families. In: Burden N, DeFazio Quinn D, O'Brien D, et al, editors. Ambulatory surgical nursing. 2nd edition. Philadelphia: WB Saunders; 2000. p. 639.

to a pediatric floor in the hospital [24]. Factors that may influence discharge are administration of medications, extubation time, ability to urinate and ambulate, fluid intake, and control of postoperative nausea and vomiting. Many facilities now discharge children without these requirements provided they are addressed in written discharge instructions.

Written discharge instructions should complement verbal instructions and teaching given by the PACU nurse. These instructions serve as a reference for the parents as they care for their child at home. Telephone numbers are included with specific instructions in case an emergency occurs after discharge.

QUALITY IMPROVEMENT/RESEARCH

Quality improvement processes should be used to obtain feedback from children and parents to ensure that intended outcomes of preoperative teaching, preadmission preparation, age-specific care, and appropriate pain management were achieved. Nursing routines, procedures, and teaching must be continually validated and altered by documented research [20]. Because of the large numbers of patients and their various ages and diagnoses, the pediatric population is a valuable resource for systematic investigation that will ultimately improve care for all children and translate into evidence-based practice.

SUMMARY

Care of the pediatric patient throughout the surgical process continues to grow and develop. This article attempts to address the special needs of the pediatric population from the preoperative period through postanesthesia. Integrating the psychosocial, developmental, and cognitive domains of the child is of the utmost importance [34]. The family (parents and child) must be cared for equally because caring for only one part of the family unit fails both.

The framework for delivery of nursing care is built on the ANA Standards of Maternal and Child Health Nursing and Pediatric Clinical Nursing Practice, AORN Standards and Recommended Practices, and the ASPAN Standards of Perianesthesia Nursing. The nursing process serves as the practice model.

The perioperative/perianesthesia team must work together to provide a plan of care for the pediatric patient that centers on effective preoperative preparation, dedicated delivery of care, and prevention of physiologic and behavioral problems [35]. When the nurses, family, and child all work together to achieve these goals, desired patient outcomes are accomplished and satisfaction is achieved.

Further readings

Bates T, Broome M. Preparation of children for hospitalization and surgery: a review of the literature. J Pediatr Nurs 1986;1:230–9.

Hoffman WD, Natanson C. Pulmonary complications of anesthesia. In: Rogers MC, Tinker JH, Covino BG, et al, editors. Principles and practice of anesthesiology. St. Louis (MO): Mosby; 1993.

Mansson ME, Fredrikzon B, Rosberg B. Comparison of preparation and narcotic-sedative premedication in children undergoing surgery. Pediatr Nurs 1992;18:337–42.

References

[1] American Nurses Association. Position statement in standards of maternal child health nursing practice. Kansas City (MO): Congress of Nursing Practice/ANA; 1983/1995.

[2] Swearingen PL. All-in-one care planning resource. St Louis (MO): Mosby; 2004.

[3] Ireland D. Pediatric patients and their families. In: Burden N, DeFazio Quinn D, O'Brien D, et al, editors. Ambulatory surgical nursing. 2nd edition. Philadelphia: Saunders; 2000. p. 613–42.

[4] Phillips N. Berry and Kohn's operating room technique. 2nd edition. St Louis (MO): Mosby; 2004.

[5] Hockenberry MJ, Wilson D, Winkelstein ML, et al. Wong's nursing care of infants and children. 7th edition. St. Louis (MO): Elsevier; 2003.

[6] Joint Commission on Accreditation of Healthcare Organization. Comprehensive accreditation manual for hospitals: the official handbook (CAMH). Chicago: Joint Commission on Accreditation of Healthcare Organization; 2001.

[7] Betz CL, Sowden LA. Mosby's pediatric nursing reference. 4th edition. St. Louis (MO): Mosby; 2000.

[8] Dresser S, Melnyk BM. The effectiveness of conscious sedation on anxiety, pain, and procedural complications in young children. Pediatr Nurs 2003;29(4):320–32.

[9] Williams C, Davis CM. Therapeutic interaction in nursing. Sudbury (MA): Jones & Bartlett; 2005.

[10] Hannallah RS. Pediatric anesthesia in the community hospital. ASA Newsletter 2000;64(2): 1–4.

[11] Rankin SH, Stallings KD, London F. Patient education in health and illness. 5th edition. Philadelphia: Lippincott Williams & Wilkins; 2004.

[12] Iwinski S. Preoperative fasting (NPO): guidelines for breastfed infants and children. Available at: http://www.lalecheleague.org/llleaderweb/LV/LVDDecJan02p132.html. August 15, 2005.

[13] Maltby JR, Chir B. Update in anesthesia: (ASA) fasting guidelines. Available at: http://www.nda.ox.ac.uk/wfsa/html/u12/u1202_02.htm. August 15, 2005.

[14] DeFazio-Quinn D. The pediatric patient. In: DeFazio-Quinn D, Schick L, editors. Perianesthesia nursing core curriculum. 2nd edition. Philadelphia: Saunders; 2004. p. 138–79.

[15] American Academy of Pediatrics Committee on Drugs. Guidelines for monitoring and management of pediatric patients during and after sedation for diagnostic and therapeutic procedures: addendum. Pediatrics 2002;110(4):836–8.

[16] Maldonado SS, LeBoeuf MB. Pediatric surgery. In: Rothrock JC, editor. Alexander's care of the patient in surgery. 12th edition. St. Louis (MO): Mosby; 2003. p. 1211–93.

[17] Goel S. Pediatric anesthesia. Available at: www.pediatriconcall.com. August 15, 2005.

[18] Popovich DM, Richiuson N, Danck G. Pediatric healthcare provider's knowledge of pulse oximetry. Pediatr Nurs 2004;30(1):14–20.

[19] American Society of Perianesthesia Nurses. Standards of perianesthesia nursing. Cherry Hill (NJ): American Society of Perianesthesia Nurses; 2004.

[20] Board R, Ryan-Wenger N. Stressors and stress symptoms of mothers with children in the PACU. J Pediatr Nurs 2003;18(3):195–202.

[21] Johnson D. Care of the pediatric patient. In: Drain C, editor. Perianesthesia nursing: a critical approach. Philadelphia: Saunders; 2003. p. 661–81.

[22] Morgan G, Mikhail M, Murray M. Clinical anesthesiology. 3rd edition. New York: Lang; 2002.

[23] Litman RS. Pediatric anesthesia—the requisites. St. Louis (MO): Elsevier; 2004.

[24] DeSoto H. Management dilemmas of pediatric patients. In: Twersky RS, editor. The ambulatory anesthesia handbook. St. Louis (MO): Mosby; 1995. p. 145.

[25] Gregory GA. Pediatric anesthesia. 4th edition. St. Louis (MO): Churchill-Livingstone/Elsevier; 2002.

[26] Litman RS, Rosenberg H. Malignant hyperthermia. Available at: http://www. medscape.com. August 15, 2005.

[27] Hopkins P. Malignant hyperthermia: advances in clinical management and diagnosis. Br J Anaesth 2000;85(1):118–28.

[28] McCaffery M, Pasero C. Pain clinical manual. 2nd edition. Philadelphia (PA): Mosby; 1999. p. 63.

[29] Beyer J. Judging the effectiveness of analgesia for children with sickle cell Disease. J Pain Symptom Manage 2000;19:63–72.

[30] Luffy R, Grove SK. Examining the validity, reliability, and preference of three pediatric pain measurement tools in African-American children. Pediatr Nurs 2003;29:54–9.

[31] Beyer J, Turner SB, Jones L, et al. The alternate forms reliability of the Oucher pain scale. Pain Manag Nurs 2005;6(1):10–7.

[32] Helgadóttir HL, Wilson ME. Temperament and pain in 3 to 7-year old children undergoing tonsillectomy. J Pediatr Nurs 2004;19(3):204–13.

[33] Helgadóttir HL. Pain management practices in children after surgery. J Pediatr Nurs 2000;15(5):334–40.

[34] Wollin SR, Plummer JL, Owen H, et al. Anxiety in children having elective surgery. J Pediatr Nurs 2004;19(2):128–32.

[35] Hatfield NT, Broadribb V. Broadribb's introductory pediatric nursing. 6th edition. Philadelphia: Lippincott Williams & Wilkins; 2003.

Nurs Clin N Am 41 (2006) 299–311

NURSING CLINICS
OF NORTH AMERICA

Management of the Special Needs of the Pregnant Surgical Patient

Sharon Romanoski, RN, MBA, CNOR, RNFA

Paoli Hospital, 255 West Lancaster Avenue, Paoli, PA 19355, USA

MANAGEMENT OF THE SPECIAL NEEDS OF THE PREGNANT SURGICAL PATIENT

Fewer than 1% of women undergo surgery during pregnancy, but those who do present unique challenges to the perioperative nurse and entire surgical team [1]. Each patient requires the services of a multidisciplinary team, including the surgeon, obstetric anesthesia providers, perioperative and obstetrical nurses, and possibly a neonatologist, depending on the patient's stage of pregnancy [2].

PHYSIOLOGIC CHANGES IN MOTHER AND FETUS

The physiologic changes that occur in women and the needs of the fetus during various stages of development impact the care that the surgical team delivers to the pregnant patient. Each stage of pregnancy presents different concerns that must be addressed in the care of the mother and baby.

In the first trimester, implantation of the embryo and development of the fetus occur. The limbs and the circulatory, nervous, and respiratory systems develop during this time. The beginnings of most of these systems occur by the end of the eighth week, and by the end of the twelfth week the sex of the baby can be distinguished on ultrasound. During the second and third trimesters the fetus continues to develop, mature all systems, and gain weight in preparation for delivery [3].

The pregnant woman's body adapts in a profound way to the demands of the fetus throughout pregnancy. During the first trimester as the embryo implants, the placenta enlarges and secretes massive amounts of hormones. These hormones have the effect of stopping further ovulation and safeguarding the pregnancy until delivery. The uterus softens and enlarges so that by the end of the first trimester, the gravid uterus can no longer be contained within the pelvis. As the uterus continues to enlarge it rotates to the right and displaces the intestines higher into the abdominal cavity, eventually encroaching on the liver. This displacement increases the risk for esophageal reflex after about

E-mail address: RomanoskiS@MLHS.org

0029-6465/06/$ – see front matter
doi:10.1016/j.cnur.2006.01.009

18 to 20 weeks. The maternal blood volume increases about 45% during the course of the pregnancy, thus increasing cardiac output appreciably [3]. The clotting factors in the blood and the volume of plasma increase, causing a decrease in the blood hemoglobin level. As the uterus increases in size, it can compress the vena cava and aorta when the woman lies in the supine position [3].

COMMON CONDITIONS THAT REQUIRE SURGERY DURING PREGNANCY

Surgery of any kind presents a risk to mother and fetus. Therefore, all elective surgery should be postponed until the delivery. All women of childbearing age should have a serum pregnancy test during preadmission testing to rule out pregnancy before commencing with elective surgery [4]. However, emergency surgery should never be postponed once a definitive diagnosis has been made, because the risks to mother and child are far greater if the condition is left untreated. Common emergency surgery involves trauma, appendicitis, and intestinal obstruction. All of these conditions are potentially life-threatening and require immediate surgery. Common urgent conditions include cholecystitis, urinary calculi, malignancies, and orthopedic emergencies (eg, fractures, herniated intervertebral discs, ligament tears). Many of these conditions can be managed conservatively and surgery can occur after delivery [5–7].

TIMING THE SURGICAL PROCEDURE—RISKS INVOLVED

The best time to perform surgery during pregnancy is the second trimester. By this time the major systems of the fetus are formed, thus decreasing the risk for fetal malformations caused by the use of anesthetic agents. Although for ethical reasons drugs are never tested on pregnant women, retrospective studies on thousands of women who underwent surgery during the first trimester of pregnancy have shown no statistical difference in congenital malformations compared with women who had not undergone surgery [1]. Nonetheless, the theoretical risk still exists until after the twelfth week of pregnancy. The uterus has not enlarged enough to infringe on the abdominal structures of the mother so that manipulation of the uterus during abdominal surgery can be kept to a minimum (Fig. 1).

Surgical patients have a 12% rate of spontaneous abortion during the first trimester. This rate drops to 0% to 5.6% during the second trimester [5]. Whether this reduction is caused by the underlying condition, the surgery itself, or anesthesia is unclear. This event is most common during abdominal surgery. Surgery during the third trimester carries a higher rate of preterm labor and low birth weight babies. The increased size of the gravid uterus together with the hypercoagulable state of pregnancy predisposes to varicose veins, edema, and thromboembolic complications after surgery, particularly in open abdominal surgery.

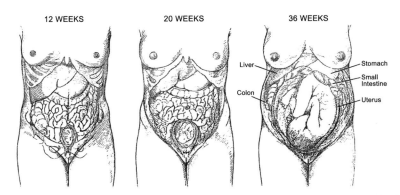

Fig. 1. Enlargement of the uterus to accommodate the developing fetus shifts intra-abdominal contents superiorly and compresses retroperitoneal structures. These effects are particularly important during the second and third trimesters. (*From* ACS Surgery. Principles and practice—the pregnant surgical patient. Available at: www.acssurgery.com/acsonline/chapters/ch803.htm; with permission.) Accessed August 8, 2005.

ANESTHESIA CONSIDERATIONS

Most pregnant patients presenting for surgery are young healthy patients outside of the immediate disease process. The choice of anesthetic agents depends on the location of the surgical site and the stage of pregnancy. During the first trimester, regional blocks or spinal anesthesia may be preferable to general anesthesia to minimize fetal exposure to medications. However, if general anesthesia is required, the lowest effective dose of medication should be used. The administration of nitrous oxide and benzodiazopams should be avoided during the first trimester of pregnancy because of their teratogenic effects [1]. Preoxygenation and administration of high concentrations of oxygen during the procedure are essential to the prevention of fetal desaturation. Cricoid pressure should be considered during the induction of general anesthesia to prevent aspiration of gastric contents, which is caused by the increased emptying time and decreased tone of the gastroesophageal sphincter until the endotracheal tube has been inserted and stabilized. The patient should not be placed in the dorsal recumbent position but in a slight left lateral position either by placing a wedge under the patient's right side or airplaning the operating room bed laterally to take the weight of the uterus off the aorta and vena cava [6]. usual, blood pressure, temperature, oxygen saturation, and carbon dioxide must be monitored during the entire procedure. During laparotomy the anesthesia provider should supply sufficient relaxation to prevent uterine contractions in the event any intra-abdominal manipulation occurs.

Fetal monitoring should be performed during any procedure involving a viable fetus. However, controversy surrounds the issue of fetal heart rate and uterine contractions on the previable fetus. Obstetricians do not feel that fetal monitoring is necessary for previable fetuses because a Cesarean section would not be performed anyway [4]. However, anesthesiologists contend that monitoring even a previable fetus is valuable so that they can take action to preserve fetal well-being if a change from the baseline rate occurs. In his article "Anesthesia during non-obstetric surgery," Penning [4] contends that the "fetal heart rate and uterine contraction monitoring can be useful and should not be reserved for viable pregnancies only." Fetal monitoring is not useful before 18 weeks and is generally most useful beyond 22 weeks. At emergence, the anesthesia provider should wait until the patient is fully awake before extubation, and fetal monitoring should continue into the recovery area for 12 to 24 hours postoperatively [4,7].

PERIOPERATIVE NURSING CARE—ASSOCIATION OF PERIOPERATIVE NURSING STANDARDS

The perioperative nurse must develop an individualized care plan that considers all aspects of the patient's history [8,9]. The assessment includes the patient's health history; specific diagnosis; stage of fetal development; current comorbid conditions; current medications; and allergies, particularly to latex. The nurse must ascertain that an obstetric consultation has been performed and that the role of the obstetrician has been determined. In most settings this documentation occurs in a preoperative holding area, the patient floor, or the emergency department. The nurse should review the data and laboratory tests and communicate all pertinent information to the surgeon, anesthesia provider, and other members of the surgical team. These data are used to establish nursing diagnoses for the patient.

Nursing diagnoses address conditions for which the surgical patient is at risk that can be managed through nursing interventions. One example is the potential for high anxiety caused by patient concern about not only her own condition but also the potential negative effects on her unborn child. Other possible diagnoses could include the risk for chemical and thermal burns caused by preparatory solutions; hypothermia; injury caused by positioning; infection; and retained foreign bodies [9].

After establishing the nursing diagnoses, the nurse must identify the expected outcomes of surgical nursing care. Among these would be the absence of infection, retained foreign bodies, damage to skin integrity caused by positioning, and hypothermia, and the reduction of anxiety. To attain these results the nurse must devise a plan that incorporates all nursing diagnoses, expected outcomes, and safe practices during the surgical procedure [9]. A comprehensive nursing care plan should provide for

- Patient identification and confirmation of the planned surgery
- Appropriate instruments and equipment for planned and unplanned events
- Environmental monitoring (eg, temperature, humidity, traffic)
- Aseptic technique
- Medications for the anesthesia provider and the surgical field
- Collaboration of care among departments (eg, obstetrics for fetal monitoring, radiology for intraoperative ultrasound)
- Updating the family of the patient's progress

The perioperative nurse should also plan to alert nurses who will be caring for the patient after surgery in the postanesthesia care department or intensive care unit (ICU).

IMPLEMENTATION OF THE NURSING CARE PLAN

Patient identification requires the nurse to check the armband and receive verbal verification from the patient. Two forms of identification should be confirmed, such as birth date or medical record number plus the patient's name. Verification of the planned surgery and any known allergies occurs at this time. Once the patient has been moved to the operating room bed and anesthesia has been induced, the care providers must take a "time out" to agree on the patient identification and planned surgery [10]. Confirmation of planned surgery must include surgical side or site if, for example, the condition is an ovarian torsion or hydronephrosis.

The nurse must provide appropriate instrumentation and supplies for the anticipated surgery, including medications, preparatory solutions, sterile supplies, and instrument trays. The surgical team must count all sponges, sharps, and instruments according to hospital policy and document them on the patient record [8]. Adherence to sterile technique throughout the surgery requires that any breaks in technique must be reported and corrected.

PROVIDING MEDICATIONS

Local anesthetics and antibiotics may be needed during the procedure. The nurse must be aware of the effects of the medications and any possible effects on the developing fetus.

Different medications pose different risks during the various stages of pregnancy. In 1979 the US Food and Drug Administration published a classification for drug safety during pregnancy, provided in Box 1. However, this classification applies only to the first trimester of pregnancy during which fetal systems are forming.

Box 1: US Food and Drug Administration Classification for Drug Safety

Category A: Drugs that have been found safe in controlled studies on pregnant women.

Category B: Drugs that either have animal studies that show no fetal damage but have no human studies, or show ill effects in animals but not in human studies.

Category C: Drugs that either have no animal or human studies or have studies that show adverse effects on the fetus with no available data on human subjects.

Category D: Drugs that show some fetal risk but have benefits that are believed to outweigh the risks.

Category X: Drugs with proven risks to the fetus which outweigh the benefits and should not be used under any circumstances [3].

Table 1 addresses some of the medications more commonly used during pregnancy. Most local anesthetics such as lidocaine and bupivacaine have been shown to be safe.

PATIENT PREPARATION

Before anesthesia is induced during surgery, the perioperative nurse must apply antiembolism stockings or sequential compression devices (SCDs) to prevent emboli during the surgery. During induction of anesthesia the nurse might provide cricoid pressure as the anesthesia provider intubates the patient. A Foley catheter is then inserted to measure urinary output intraoperatively and keep the bladder decompressed to prevent inadvertent injury. The dispersive pad for the electrosurgery device should be placed as close to the surgical site as possible, while carefully avoiding bony prominences. Padding should be placed around the area of the skin to be prepared for incision to prevent pooling of solutions under the patient. These absorbent pads should be removed before sterile drapes are applied.

During the procedure, the perioperative nurse monitors the conditions in the room, obtains necessary surgical supplies, operates equipment such as lasers and video systems, and maintains communications with the family and the patient's obstetrician as needed. Obstetric nurses who may be unfamiliar with the operating room environment are responsible for performing the fetal monitoring. The circulating nurse must assist the obstetric nurse as needed. The perioperative nurse also participates in sponge, sharps, and instrument counts. Counts may need to be suspended in extreme emergencies. Each institution should develop policies that document these events and provide for appropriate follow-up, such as abdominal radiograph when feasible, depending on the patient's condition [8]. After wound closure the nurse provides necessary dressings and assists the anesthesia provider during emergence. The nurse then

Medication	FDA classification	Effects on fetus
Table 1		
Medications commonly used during surgery		
Local anesthetics		
Lidocaine (Xylocaine)	B	Usually safe
Bipuvicaine (Marcaine)	C	May cause bradycardia
Antibiotics		
Penicillins	B	Safe
Cephalosporins	B	Safe
Metronidazole (Flagyl)	B	Use after 1st trimester only
Quinolones	C	Affects fetal bone and cartilage
Vancomycin	C	Ototoxicity and nephrotoxicity
Gentamycin	C	Possible ototoxicity
Clindamycin	B	No known problems

Modified from Parungo CP, Brooks DC. The pregnant surgical patient [ACS Surgery-Web site]. Available at: www.acssurgery.com/acsonline/chapters/ch803.htm. Accessed August 8, 2005.

assists with moving the patient safely to a bed or stretcher and accompanies the patient to the postanesthesia recovery area.

EVALUATION OF NURSING CARE

Once in the recovery room, the perioperative nurse reports patient status and surgical outcomes to the perianesthesia nurse and evaluates the results of the nursing care. Absence of chemical and burns from the electrosurgical pad, skin conditions after positioning and preparation, and any other relevant observations should be documented. If fetal monitoring occurred during the procedure, an obstetric nurse will continue to do so in the postanesthesia care unit (PACU). The patient must be closely monitored in the postoperative period for signs of spontaneous abortion, such as bleeding and cramping. Any remaining issues, such as anxiety, knowledge deficits, or pain control, must be audited postoperatively through patient visits and consultation with the primary care nurses, obstetrician, and family members. Retrospective chart audits will reveal issues such as postoperative infections that cannot be readily evaluated immediately after surgery.

NURSING CONSIDERATIONS FOR SPECIFIC PROCEDURES

Trauma

Trauma is the leading cause of maternal death in this country, accounting for 46.3%. Motor vehicle accidents account for 55% to 60% of trauma in pregnant women, followed by falls (22%) and domestic violence (21%) [5]. Blunt abdominal trauma, most often associated with motor vehicle accidents, causes more harm to the mother than the fetus, whereas direct penetrating injuries such as gunshot wounds or stabbings are more often fatal to the fetus than to the mother. Placental abruption occurs in 40% to 66% of major trauma victims, but often occurs only after definitive surgery. These patients are best cared for in a regional trauma center where trauma surgeons, obstetricians specializing in high-risk pregnancies, and specially trained obstetric nurses are available. After the woman has been stabilized in the emergency department, she will be transferred to the operating room for exploratory laparotomy or chest surgery to control bleeding and repair any visceral damage [11,12].

Depending on the gestational age of the fetus, a multidisciplinary team, including the surgeon, obstetrician, anesthesiologist, and nursing staff (both perioperative and obstetric), must be present during the surgery. As the nurse prepares for exploratory laparotomy, instrumentation for vascular surgery, bowel surgery, and a possible Cesarean section must be made available. Placental abruption (abruptio-placenta) is life-threatening to the mother and could cause death from blood loss if the situation occurs during the second or third trimester of pregnancy. Little time for assessment may be available before surgery, so speed and efficiency is paramount in salvaging the life of the mother and baby. The nurse must reassure the patient that everything possible will be done to save her baby, but no promises should be made.

If the patient is unstable, priority is given to immediate anesthesia and open surgery. Positioning is especially important in this situation. The patient is placed in a modified left lateral position after 20 weeks gestation because the patient's circulatory system is already compromised by the traumatic event. The insertion of a Foley catheter and application of SCDs are also important. The circulating nurse is responsible for delivering supplies to the surgical field; arranging for blood and laboratory work to be performed during surgery; obtaining blood and intravenous fluids for the anesthesiologist; conducting sponge, sharps, and instrument counts with the scrub person; and communicating with the family as the surgery progresses. The circulating registered nurse is also responsible for ensuring the immediate availability of the crash cart. If fetal demise occurs from the traumatic incident, the nurse should arrange for a bereavement counselor or spiritual advisor to support the patient and family if the desire for this intervention is expressed and the patient is hemodynamically stable. If the patient is still unstable as surgery concludes, the nurse should offer emotional support to the family and arrange for any help the family requests. The patient will be transferred to an ICU for close observation after surgery. In addition to the normal intensive nursing care, obstetric nurses will be on hand to monitor the patient closely for signs of abruptio-placenta well into the postoperative period. Perioperative nurses must be alert for an emergency Cesarean section if this occurs.

Appendicitis and Intestinal Obstruction

Appendicitis is the most common surgical problem in pregnant women. Approximately 1 case per 550 pregnancies has been documented nationally [13]. It occurs at the same frequency in pregnant women as it does in nonpregnant women. Once diagnosis has been confirmed, surgery must be performed immediately regardless of the stage of pregnancy because delay can result in catastrophic perforation and peritonitis. Appendicitis treated immediately has a 2% to 8% incidence of fetal loss, which rises as high as 35% if rupture and peritonitis are present [5]. Intestinal obstruction usually of the small bowel rarely occurs in women of child-bearing age. Adhesions from previous surgery and volvulus account for 80% of all obstructions [5]. Incidence of fetal mortality rises when patients have a history of abdominal surgery with adhesions.

Appendectomy is usually a routine procedure even in pregnant patients and generally requires limited instrumentation and a small incision. Appendectomy can be performed with sedation and local anesthesia alone. Bowel obstructions require full laparotomy instrumentation, including larger retractors and gastrointestinal stapling devices. Specific nursing concerns vary with the stage of fetal development, but culture media must be available in the event of perforation. The surgeon usually wishes to irrigate with warmed antibiotic solutions and may leave a drain in the patient. Fetal monitoring and consultation with obstetric nurses must be performed according to the established protocols. A continuum of care must be established to monitor the patient for signs of fetal distress in the postoperative period. If peritonitis is present the patient might need to be transferred to the ICU for observation. The perioperative nurse is responsible for making those arrangements. The patient and her family will be very anxious about the effect of the surgery on her baby, and all efforts should be made to allay their fears.

Gallbladder Disease (Cholecystitis, Cholelithiasis)

The increase in progesterone during pregnancy decreases the motility of the gallbladder, delaying emptying. Consequently, the risk for gallstones increases in pregnancy, making acute cholecystitis the second most common surgical disease in pregnant women [2,4,14]. Most physicians prefer to treat these patients conservatively and avoid surgery during pregnancy if possible. However, surgery becomes necessary in 25% of patients because of recurrent symptoms, gangrene, or perforation of the gallbladder [2]. The best time to operate is the second trimester if the patient's condition permits. Laparoscopic cholecystectomy is generally the preferred method for gallbladder surgery. Numerous studies have shown that laparoscopy is as safe for pregnant women as laparotomy and has several advantages [15,16].

Laparoscopy is performed through small incisions that allow decreased bowel manipulation, which in turn reduces the risk for adhesions. Early ambulation and a reduced requirement for pain medication decreases the risk for thromboembolism and fetal depression caused by the use of narcotics. Laparoscopy does not have an increased rate of spontaneous abortion or preterm delivery compared with open laparotomy, and it can be safely performed throughout pregnancy. However, if the enlarged uterus makes laparoscopic surgery impossible, then an open cholecystectomy must be performed [4]. The greatest identified risks from laparoscopy are damage to the uterus caused by insertion of the insufflation needle; fetal hypoxia or hypercapnia as a result of carbon dioxide insufflation; and decreased uterine blood flow caused by increased intra-abdominal pressure [4,15,16]. These hazards can be modified by maintaining intra-abdominal pressure below 15 mm Hg, positioning the patient in modified left lateral position, and using an open technique to insert the primary trocar. Fetal monitoring during this procedure is essential [16].

Perioperative nurses must be familiar with the video systems used in laparoscopic surgery, particularly the carbon dioxide insufflator. The circulating nurse is responsible for ensuring that the flow rate is adjusted to an appropriate setting. Maternal and fetal safety take precedence over surgeon preference in these instances. Other important considerations for these patients are the application of SCDs, insertion of the Foley catheter, and positioning of the patient for optimum exposure while avoiding impingement of the uterus on the great vessels of the abdomen. The obstetric nurse might need assistance with fetal monitoring. Arrangements may need to be made for blood work, such as hemoglobin and hematocrit or arterial blood gasses. Because the laparoscopic procedure may need to be converted to an open procedure, the nurse should be prepared to convert swiftly and efficiently.

Laparoscopy could also be used for appendectomy or ovarian torsion during pregnancy. Nursing considerations would be similar to those for laparoscopic cholecystectomy.

Hydronephrosis, Renal Colic, Urinary Calculi

Renal colic is the most common reason for admitting the pregnant female to the hospital. Hydronephrosis in some degree is present in 90% of all pregnant women [17,18]. Pregnant women are no more likely to form ureteral or renal calculi than nonpregnant women, and most calculi that form pass with conservative treatment. However, about 1 in 1500 patients develop stones that produce hydronephrosis, infection, flank pain, and hematuria [17]. The patient who has untreated obstruction combined with infection has a high risk for spontaneous abortion and premature labor. An accurate diagnosis must be definitively established. MRI is proving to be the modality of choice for diagnosing obstruction in the pregnant patient [17].

In normal circumstances the treatment of choice for kidney stones is extracorporeal shock wave lithotripsy. This procedure is contraindicated in pregnancy because the effect of the treatment on the fetus is unknown. Relief of the pain and hydronephrosis can be accomplished by inserting a ureteral stent immediately and reserving definitive treatment of the stone until after delivery. Cystoscopy and ureteral stent insertion can be performed using ultrasonography instead of fluoroscopy for stent placement. Once symptoms are relieved, the patient may return home. The stent may need to be changed monthly on an outpatient basis until delivery because calcium deposits tend to collect along the stent's length. Ureteral stones may be treated with ureteroscopy and stone removal by basket, or laser lithotripsy can be used safely under direct vision [17].

Primary nursing considerations for these patients are positioning, fluid irrigation, and the prevention of emboli and infection. Cystoscopy is performed in the lithotomy position, and may occur in a specially designed cystoscopy suite or main operating room on a standard operating room bed adapted for cystoscopy. The perioperative nurse must be familiar with the operation and set up of OR beds and the equipment used. Some institutions use ultrasound technicians from the radiology department and some have their own ultrasound machine in the unit. The perioperative nurse must coordinate the use of this equipment with the various departments involved. A separate laser nurse or technician must operate the laser according to institutional policy if laser lithotripsy is performed. SCDs must be applied before positioning the patient's legs in stirrups on the urology table. A wedge or sandbag must be placed under the patient's right side to displace the weight of the uterus. Many of these procedures are performed using light intravenous sedation with a local anesthetic to allow access to the urethra. The patient remains aware of her environment, so the circulating nurse must maintain a calm environment. The patient must be cautioned to report any return of symptoms to her physician. The patient will generally be placed on antibiotics to ward off infection.

Cesarean Section

The definitive surgery for pregnant women is the Cesarean delivery, usually referred to as *C-section*. Elective (occurring before labor) C-sections increased nearly 44% from 1994 to 2001. In 2003 nearly 28% of all infants born were delivered through C-section [19]. Box 2 lists the 12 indications for C-section.

Although repeat C-sections and breech deliveries are easily scheduled, other indications may occur urgently during labor. In many institutions the Cesarean births occur in the maternity department rather than in the main operating suite, but the principles of perioperative nursing remain the same. Nurses must prepare a set of instruments for the C-section. A neonatologist or neonatal nurse practitioner will be available to care for the baby immediately after delivery and therefore a warming crib and resuscitative equipment must be available in the operating room.

Emotional support is extremely necessary for women undergoing C-section because they are concerned about the well-being of their baby, particularly if the procedure is being performed on an urgent basis. The mother will have a regional anesthetic without sedation to prevent sedation of the infant. This method also affords the parents the opportunity to share in the experience of birth. The husband or significant other will usually be present and should be encouraged to support his wife as she undergoes the surgery. The whole team should provide a family-oriented experience for the couple as their baby is born. The mother will be lying in the supine position with a rolled towel or large bag of irrigating solution under her right side to lift the baby off her vena cava and aorta. The nurse will insert a Foley catheter to empty the bladder and protect it from injury during the surgery. Because the uterus is a hollow organ capable of harboring a foreign body, an additional sponge, sharps, and instrument count must be performed before closure of the uterus

---

Box 2: The 12 indications for Cesarean Section

- Improved fetal monitoring
- Increased first-time pregnancies
- Increased age of pregnant women
- Malpresentation of the fetus (such as breech presentation)
- Antepartum bleeding (bleeding during pregnancy)
- Hypertension
- Increasing malpractice litigation
- Repeat C-sections
- Failure of fetus to progress
- Fetal distress
- Macrosomia (fetus is too large)
- Maternal soft tissue disorder

immediately after the baby and placenta are delivered. The other two counts should be performed as usual during closure of the abdomen [8].

After the neonate has been examined, and depending on the stability of mother and baby, the bonding process may proceed by allowing the parents to cradle the infant. Many of today's maternity departments are family-centered environments with labor, delivery, and postpartum care all performed in one room involving the same nurses. In this case, the parents and baby are roomed together and cared for by the nurse who assisted with the infant at delivery. In other facilities the mother and baby are returned to the mother's room and recovered by the maternity nurses who cared for the mother while she was in labor or who admitted her for her scheduled C-section. Patients who required general anesthesia are taken to PACU for recovery and the infant is transferred to the nursery at least temporarily.

SUMMARY

The perioperative nurse might interact with pregnant patients who undergo procedures such as breast biopsy, fracture management, or head and neck surgery for a malignant process. Fortunately these instances are rare. The nursing care for these patients would be similar to that for a nonpregnant person, while considering factors of gestational age and maternal physiologic and psychologic change. Every pregnant patient deserves a multidisciplinary team, a defined plan of care, and communication among all members. Each surgery requires unique preparation and uses different skills by the perioperative nurse. The importance of strict adherence to asepsis, attention to patient safety, and emotional support cannot be overstressed. The goal of the perioperative nurse must always be to provide exceptional care to every patient and to assure the best outcome possible for the patient and unborn child.

Acknowledgments

Alex Anthopoulos, MD, Obstetrician-Gynecologist, Paoli Hospital, Paoli, PA; James R. Bollinger, MD, Chief of Urology, Paoli Hospital, Paoli, PA; David Robinson, MD, Staff Anesthesiologist, Paoli Hospital, Paoli, PA; and Mojdeh Saberin-Williams, MD, Obstetrician-Gynecologist, Paoli Hospital, Paoli, PA.

References

[1] Chestnut DH. Obstetric anesthesia: principles and practice. 3rd edition. St. Louis (MO): Mosby; 2004.

[2] Committee on Obstetrical Practice. Nonobstetric surgery in pregnancy. Compendium of selected publications. Washington (DC): The American College of Obstetricians and Gynecologists; 2004. p.81.

[3] Cunningham FG, Gant NF, Leveno KJ, et al. Williams obstetrics. 21st edition. New York: McGraw-Hill; 2001.

[4] Fleisher LA. Evidence-based practice of anesthesiology. 1st edition. St. Louis (MO): Elsevier; 2004. p.18–21.

[5] Parungo CP, Brooks DC. The pregnant surgical patient. ACS surgery: principles and practice, section 9. Available at: www.acssurgery.com/acsonline/chapters/ch803.htm. Accessed August 8, 2005.

[6] Phillips N. Berry & Kohn's operating room technique. 10th edition. St. Louis (MO): Mosby; 2004.
[7] Bready LL, Mullins RM, Noorily SH, et al. Decision making in anesthesiology. St. Louis (MO): Mosby; 2000.
[8] AORN. Standards, recommended practices, and guidelines. Denver (CO): The Association; 2005.
[9] Swearingen PL. All-in-one care planning resource. St. Louis (MO): Mosby; 2004.
[10] JCAHO. Universal protocol for preventing wrong site, wrong procedure, wrong person surgery, 1993. Available at: http://www.jcaho.org/accredited+organizations/patient+safety/universal+protocol/universal_protocol. Accessed August 8, 2005.
[11] Committee on Obstetrical Practice. Obstetric aspects of trauma management. Compendium of selected publications. Washington (DC): The American College of Obstetricians and Gynecologists; 2004. p.197–203.
[12] Grossman NB. Blunt trauma in pregnancy. Am Fam Physician 2004;70(7):1303–10.
[13] Angelini DJ. Obstetric Triage revisited: update on non-obstetric surgical conditions in pregnancy. J Midwifery Womens Health 2003;48(2):111–8.
[14] Cordero SB. Your patient has cholecystitis and she's pregnant. Nursing 2002;32(11):1–4.
[15] Fatum M, Nathan R. Laparoscopic surgery during pregnancy. In Obstetrical and Gynecological Survey, 56(1): 50–59, 2001. Available at: http://www.obgynsurvey.com/pt/re/obgynsurv/fulltext.00006254-20. Accessed August 8, 2005.
[16] SAGES Committee on Standards of Practice. SAGES guidelines for laparoscopic surgery during pregnancy. Available at: http://www.sages.org/sagespublication.php?doc=23. Accessed August 8, 2005.
[17] Choe JM, Prasad R. Pregnancy and urolithiasis, Available at: Emedicine.com. Accessed August 8, 2005.
[18] Rothrock JC. Alexander's care of the patient in surgery. 12th edition. St. Louis (MO): Mosby; 2003.
[19] Hitti M. Elective Ceasarean section deliveries rising. Available at: http://www.webmd.com/content/article/104/107595.html. Accessed August 8, 2005.

Nurs Clin N Am 41 (2006) 313–328

NURSING CLINICS
OF NORTH AMERICA

Nursing Considerations in the Geriatric Surgical Patient: the Perioperative Continuum of Care

Myrna Eileen Mamaril, MS, RN, CPAN, CAPA

University of Colorado Hospital, 4200 East Ninth Avenue, Denver, CO 80262, USA

The geriatric patient faces a myriad of issues involving: the normal aging process, altered responses to illness, surgical and anesthesia implications, appropriate surgical health care screening, focused preoperative assessments, specialized perioperative education, and comprehensive discharge planning.

The perioperative nurse's duty is to learn as much as possible about the geriatric patient through the personal interview, health history, medical record, physician consults, and testing results so that baseline health data are established and compared during all phases of the perioperative continuum, from preadmission to postanesthesia/postoperative discharge [1]. Consequently, timely communication that reports significant health care clinical findings to the appropriate health care team providers is imperative to preventing anesthesia and surgical complications. Likewise, purposeful consistent communication about the geriatric perioperative plan of care that integrates pertinent assessment information, special needs, and a dynamic nursing plan to manage actual or potential problems across the continuum of care is vital to an uneventful surgical experience and successful perioperative outcomes [2]. Although the perioperative assessment and management of older adults present unique challenges, the benefits of using a holistic, individualized approach during the surgical continuum are essential to optimal nursing care [3].

EPIDEMIOLOGY OF AGING

The population in the United States is aging at an increasing rate. Consequently, the impact on health care is profound, as a greater number of elderly patients will require anesthesia and surgery. As of 2003, people over the age of 65 years of age represented 20% of the people of the US population. This percentage is expected to increase by the year 2030 [4]. It is estimated that over one third of all surgical patients are 65 years of age or older. As life expectancy

E-mail address: myrna.mamaril@uch.edu

0029-6465/06/$ – see front matter
doi:10.1016/j.cnur.2006.01.001

of the geriatric population increases, so does the incidence of comorbidity. Comorbidity is the existence of two or more disease processes in a single individual (the patient who has hypertension and diabetes). Chronic illnesses affect recovery after anesthesia and surgery. The geriatric population consumes a disproportionate amount of health care dollars compared with the general population. Although many older adults are generally healthy, mentally astute, and self-sufficient, leading active lives into their 70s and 80s, other elderly adults are plagued with rapidly declining health, dementia, and disabilities [5]. Conversely, this disparity in elder health highlights the challenges that the nurse encounters when providing patient care.

SPECIAL CONSIDERATIONS OF OLDER ADULTS

Time is a precious in a busy surgical preparation unit [6]. Preoperative nurses must be innovative and resourceful to provide adequate time for preoperative questions and communication with their geriatric patients [5]. Sitting down, even for a brief period of time and speaking calmly in a reassuring manner establishes a therapeutic surgical milieu of mutual respect (Box 1). Creating a holistic environment of respect and caring that emphasizes an individualized approach builds an atmosphere of self-esteem and trust [3]. After all, most older adults lead productive lives and are significant members of their families and society. Aging does not mean loss of intelligence. Older adults should not be treated as children or as if they are not capable of understanding [6]. Although measures of abstract intelligence, such as mathematics, puzzle solving, or object assembling may show a decline in older adults, intelligence related to vocabulary, comprehension, and acquired information remains relatively unchanged. It may be noted, however, that intellectual changes may be attributed to declining sensory function, lessened ability to assimilate new information, and increased time requirements for processing that information [3,6].

CULTURAL PERSPECTIVE ON AGING

A culture is a set of structured social behaviors and personal beliefs that enable the individual to respond to social situations and relationships within a closed community [7]. Positive views on aging are recognized by many cultures. These aspects involve respect for the wisdom, maturity, and wealth of knowledge gained from life experiences. Ancient philosophers focused on the inner peace and understanding derived from wisdom acquired over the elderly person's lifetime. Ethnicity, culture, or social norms may influence the older adult's response to different aspects of the surgical experience, such as: trust in health care providers, acceptance of medical treatments, response to pain, and compliance with self-care activities. Cultural influences have a direct effect on the geriatric patient undergoing surgical intervention. The perioperative nurse needs to increase awareness and demonstrate sensitivity and respect when interacting with culturally diverse patients.

Box 1: Tips for effective communication with older adults

Remember:

- Sensory losses lead to frustration.
- Frustration leads to aggression or withdrawal
- Optimize sensory functioning–maximize use of hearing aids and glasses

Avoid sensory distractions such as background noise or poor lighting.

Recognize role of pain as a distraction from good communication.

Build trust; verbalize your recognition of sensory loss with patient.

Alert patient to a change in topic.

Present one point of information at a time.

Validate emotions and look for meaning behind behaviors.

Read body language and understand that body language may be altered by physical disability.

Try to see the patient's perspective.

Actively listen; give verbal or physical cues.

Ask an older adult for a summary or confirmation of instructions.

Recognize personal baggage that influences patient expectations and perspective.

Recognize cultural beliefs that influence patient's expectation.

Recognize and verbalize differing goals of patients, families, and health care professionals.

When working with interpreters, ask for translation and clearly separate agendas of family interpreter, patient, and yourself.

Try to find some common ground.

Prepared by Elaine Gould. Hartford Institute for Geriatric Nursing, Division of Nursing, New York University, April 2004; reproduced with permission.

NURSING COMPETENCY IN CARE OF THE AGING

The Atlantic Philanthropies, together with the American Nurses Association (ANA) through the American Nurses Foundation (ANF); American Nurses Credentialing Center (ANCC); and the John A. Hartford Foundation Institute for Geriatric Nursing, Division of Nursing, New York University, formed a strategic alliance in 2002. The purpose was to establish an innovative grant program to improve specialty nurses' competency in care of the aging. Over 60 national nursing specialty organizations have received these geriatric grants. Because older adults constitute the primary patient population of specialty nurses, the strategic focus is to prepare nurses in geriatrics so that ultimately the health care of older adults will improve. The goal during this 5-year award period is to infuse geriatric practice, education, and research into all areas of these specialty nursing organizations.

PREADMISSION

The preoperative or preadmission testing nurse plays a major role in establishing positive surgical outcomes. These specialty nurses use focused perioperative teaching, astute assessment skills, and keen attention to detail when reviewing the elderly patient's preoperative data, such as the history and physical examination, laboratory testing, electrocardiograph, and other pertinent information (Box 2). The preadmission nurses are the unsung heroes who are consistently under pressure to review, consult with physicians and surgeons, and ensure that all the required data are present in the medical record by

---

Box 2: Recommended health information data for preoperative evaluation

Patient information

Complete medical history and physical systems review

Complete surgical history and prior hospitalizations

Physician consults (pulmonary, cardiac, and neurologic)

Pacemaker/automatic internal cardiac defibrillator

Medical diagnosis

Proposed surgical procedure

Anesthetic history for patient and family (blood relative) with anesthesia problems

Sight, sensory, or speech impairments

Glasses/contact lenses/hearing aids

Cultural and religious beliefs

Prosthetics/dentures

Medications (prescription, over the counter, and herbal)

Height and weight

Baseline vital signs

Functional activity level

Socioeconomic issues

History of substance use (alcohol, tobacco, and recreational drugs)

Learning barriers

Mental status, competency, ability to sign surgical consent

Advanced directives

Body piercing

Family, significant other for home care support

Availability of safe transport home

Adapted from Saufl N. Preparing the elderly for surgery and anesthesia, J Perianesth Nurs 2004;12(6):372–8; with permission.

the day of surgery to prevent delays and cancellations. Imperative to the preadmission evaluation is identifying potential or actual surgical or anesthesia problems. Examples of significant clinical findings would include: difficult airways, sleep apnea, pacemakers, automatic cardiac internal defibrillators, bleeding or clotting disorders, poorly treated medical conditions, or previous anesthesia complications.

Recognizing signs and symptoms of elder abuse and reporting elder abuse are also responsibilities of the perioperative nurse. According to Koehle, there are four common categories of elder abuse: physical abuse, psychological abuse, financial abuse, and neglect [5] (Box 3). The nurse must be a patient advocate and make the appropriate referral to prevent further harm to the older adult.

AGE-RELATED RISK FACTORS

Perioperative/perianesthesia risks related to age are discussed frequently in the literature [7–9]. Advancing age should not preclude the older adult from having

---

Box 3: Elder abuse

Signs and symptoms associated with maltreatment

Patterns of health hopping (ie, relying on walk-in clinics with no regular physician follow-up)

Previous unexplained bruises or burns in unusual locations

Unexplained fractures forming recognizable patterns or shapes

Sprains or dislocations

Genital/anal bruises or bleeding

Signs of sexually transmitted diseases

Unexplained head injury

Extreme mood changes

Depression or oversedation

Lack of glasses, hearing aids, or dentures

Fearfulness

Poor personal hygiene

Malnutrition

Dehydration

Signs of confinement

Fearful of caregiver

Resource on elder abuse: http://www.gwjpan.com//NCEA

Adapted from Koehle MM. Special needs of the older adult. Ambulatory Surgical Nursing. 2000;2:646; with permission.

a successful surgery. Chronologic versus physiologic age is variable from individual to individual. Functional status refers to behaviors necessary to maintaining activities of daily living and is considered to be more important than the elderly patient's absolute age. Older adults frequently have increased comorbidities that place them at greater risk for postoperative complications. Another term, functional reserve, is often difficult to determine in the elderly, and yet it is a critical component in assessing relative risk for anesthesia and surgery.

HEALTH CARE SCREENING

Health care screening is an important assessment parameter in evaluating the health history, current medications, previous and relative anesthesia, and surgical risk the patient may encounter.

According to Pasternak, routine testing does not affect patient outcomes and is of little merit [10]. In their geriatric study, Drankic and colleagues documented the importance of the medical and surgical risk as opposed to routine testing [11]. Consequently, the evidence reveals that preoperative testing should be based on clinical history and medical and surgical risk (Tables 1, 2).

Table 1	
Potential concerns with select medication use in elderly patients	
Drug (s)	Possible concern
Trimethobenzamide	Poor efficacy, with risk of extrapyramidal symptoms
Meperidine	Not effective orally, prolonged half-life, risk of seizures due to active metabolite
Amitriptyline	High anticholinergic properties, including sedation, constipation
Ticlopidine	No better than aspirin, with safer alternatives
Ketorolac	Increase risk of bleeding in patients with asymptomatic gastrointestinal conditions
Cimetidine	Significant central nervous system effects
Long-acting benzodiazepines, such as diazepam, flurazepam, clorazepate	Prolonged sedation, increase risk of falls
Short-acting benzodiazepines in doses > lorazepam 3 mg, alprazolam 2 mg, triazolam 0.25 mg	Total daily doses should rarely exceed the maximum (due to increased sensitivity)
Diphenhydramine for sedation—use in lowest possible doses for allergic reactions only	Can cause confusion, sedation, mental status changes including delirium symptoms
Traditional nonsteroidal anti-inflammatory drugs with long half-lives (naproxen, piroxicam)	Can increase risk of gastrointestinal bleeding, acute renal failure, hypertension, and heart failure

Adapted from Kuctha A, Golembieski J. J Perianesth Nurs 2004;19(6):420; Elsevier, with permission.

Table 2
Potential concerns with select medication use in elderly patients with specific disease states

Disease state	Drugs to avoid (if possible)	Rationale
Arrhythmias	Tricyclic antidepressants	Proarrhythmic effects
Seizure	Bupropion, meperidine metabolite, clozapine, chlorpromazine, metoclopramide	Lowers seizure threshold
Hypertension	Phenylpropanolamine, amphetamines, diet pills, pseudoephedrine	May increase blood pressure
Chronic obstructive pulmonary disease	Long-acting benzodiazepines, (diazepam), nonselective beta blockers (propranolol), sedative hypnotics	May induce or exacerbate respiratory depression
Benign prostatic hypertrophy	Anticholinergics, antispasmodics, antihistamines, antidepressants opioids, muscle relaxants	May cause obstruction and impair micturition
Heart failure	Disopyramide, verapamil, high sodium content drugs	Negative inotropic effect, ability to promote water retention
Blood clotting disorders or with anticoagulants	Nonsteroidal anti-inflammatory drugs, aspirin, ticlopidine, clopidogrel, dipyridamole	Increased potential for bleeding
Chronic constipation	Tricyclic antidepressants, anticholinergics, calcium channel blockers, opioids	May worsen constipation

Adapted from Kuctha A, Golembieski J. J Perianesth Nurs 2004;19(6):420; with permission.

The American Society of Anesthesiologists has promulgated evidence-based practice guidelines for recommended preoperative testing.

POLYPHARMACY

Polypharmacy in older adults refers to taking many drugs. In addition, elderly patients may be taking herbal medicine, which further complicates the polypharmacy problem. Drug-related problems in older adults consist of therapeutic failure, adverse drug reactions, and adverse drug withdrawal events [12]. Because drug interactions are diverse, medications need to be considered carefully during the perioperative period. There are potential concerns with select medication use in geriatric patients (Tables 3, 4). Because older adults often take multiple medications and are more sensitive to adverse drug effects, they are at greater risk for drug interactions (see Tables 3, 4). Drug absorption, drug distribution, protein binding of drugs, drug elimination, and liver metabolism and renal elimination often are altered in the geriatric population, which may contribute to adverse reactions and drug interactions. The perioperative nurse needs to know how the pharmacodynamics of drug interactions affect the older adult.

Table 3
Select pharmacodynamic drug interactions

Drug A	Drug B	Effect of the interaction
Tricyclic antidepressants	Phenylephrine, pancuronium, ketamine	Hypertensive response
Diuretics that cause hypokalemia	Nondepolarizing neuromuscular blocking drugs	Prolonged neuromuscular blockade
Aminoglycoside antibiotics	Nondepolarizing neuromuscular blocking drugs	Prolonged neuromuscular blockade
Phenytoin[a], carbamazepine	Nondepolarizing neuromuscular blocking drugs (except cisatracurium)	Resistance to paralysis, ↓ duration of action
Opioids	Benzodiazepines	Additive sedation, hypnosis, respiratory depression, and hemodynamic effects
Opioids	Metoclopramide	Excessive sedation
Long-term alcohol use	Opioids	Tolerance to analgesia from opioid
Selective serotonin reuptake inhibitors (paroxetine, sertraline, fluvoxamine, fluoxetine)	Meperidine	Serotonin syndrome[b]
Monamine oxidase inhibitors	Meperidine	Severe reactions including cardiovascular instability, hyperpyrexia, seizures, coma, and possibly death
Monamine oxidase inhibitors	Dopamine, norepinephrine, epinephrine, ephedrine, phenylephrine	Risk of hypertensive crisis
Sedative–hypnotics	Alcohol	Excessive sedation
Angiotensin converting enzyme inhibitors	Nonsteroidal anti-inflammatory drugs	Hyperkalemia, reduced renal function
Antihypertensives	Vasodilators (nitroglycerin), antipsychotics, and some antidepressants	Postural hypotension
Aspirin, including low dose	Nonsteroidal anti-inflammatory drugs	Peptic ulceration
Antihypertensives	Nonsteroidal anti-inflammatory drugs	Antagonism of antihypertensive effect

Adapted from Kuctha A, Golembieski J. J Perianesth Nurs 2004;19(6):421; with permission.
[a]Chronic therapy; acute administration of a single dose can enhance neuromuscular blockade.
[b]Symptoms include mental status changes, restlessness, myoclonus, hyper-reflexia, diaphoresis, shivering, and tremor.

PHYSIOLOGY OF AGING

Perioperative and perianesthesia nurses need to understand the pathophysiologic changes that occur as a basis for signs and symptoms of the aging process. This understanding is essential to properly assess and manage the older adult

Table 4
Select pharmacokinetic drug interactions

Affected drug	Precipitant drug	Effect of the interaction
Midazolam, diazepam, clonazepam, triazolam, alprazolam	Ketoconazole, fluconazole, itraconazole, erythromycin	Excessive sedation
Alfentanil	Erythromycin	Prolonged respiratory depression
Methadone	Rifampin, phenytoin, carbamazepine, phenobarbital	Diminished analgesia, opioid withdrawal symptoms
Tricyclic antidepressants	Phenobarbital, carbamazepine, phenytoin	Reduced antidepressant effect
Tricyclic antidepressants	Cimetidine, fluoxetine, diltiazem, monoamine oxidase inhibitors	Reduced antidepressant effect
Nitrates (nitroglycerin, isosorbide mononitrate, isosorbide dinitrate)	Sildenafil, tadalafil, vardenafil	Increased hypotensive effect

Adapted from Kuctha A, Golembieski J. J Perianesth Nurs 2004;19(6):422; with permission.

perioperatively. The normal aging process is a gradual and spontaneous change that results in maturation from childhood through old age. This may refer to the common complex of diseases and impairments that are deleterious to preserving function, ultimately leading to incapacity or death. The elderly are at high risk for multiple chronic diseases, multiple drugs (polypharmacy) and the use of inappropriate drugs, uncoordinated medical care, hospitalizations, and surgery. It is imperative that perianesthesia nurses understand the physiology of aging and use critical thinking skills in assessing and managing geriatric patients' pain and comfort. According to the Emergency Nurses Association [13], "minor injuries to the elderly patient may lead to complications and a higher mortality rate due to:

- Age-related deterioration of body system function
- Decreased stress tolerance and physiologic reserve
- Greater complication risk
- Pre-existing chronic disease, particularly pulmonary and cardiovascular disease
- Pre-existing nutritional deficits"

Age-associated diseases such as diabetes, hypertension, osteoporosis, angina, peripheral vascular disease, and others cause organ systems to deteriorate over time [14,15]. The elderly are more susceptible and less tolerant of injury.

RESPIRATORY
Three dimensions affect the age-related changes in the respiratory system: aging processes, individual lifelong environmental stressors, and specific diseases that affect structural and functional components of the respiratory system.

As one ages, the extrapulmonary (musculoskeletal tissue) and intrapulmonary (lung tissue and vasculature) changes cause a decrease in the potential respiratory system expansion, ultimately altering the flow of air into and out of the lung. Osteoporosis of the ribs, hips, and vertebrae, and calcification of the costal cartilages cause increased stiffness or rigidity, decreased rib mobility, and reduced compliance of the chest wall. Furthermore, as pulmonary compliance decreases, there is also a reduction in mucociliary clearance [14]. This may be compounded by a long history of smoking, which compromises the geriatric patient exponentially. The partial pressure of oxygen decreases as much as 15% between the ages of 20 and 80 years [14]. In addition, there is less effective gas exchange at the alveolar–capillary membrane because of fewer alveoli, together with a basilar infiltration that places older patients at risk for respiratory infections. As the older adult continues to age, the chest wall experiences weaker respiratory muscles; the pulmonary system experiences a decrease in vital capacity, and the lungs lose their elasticity and become more rigid. Further complicating the respiratory function, the elderly see a degeneration of the vertebral disks that may be caused by kyphosis and scoliosis. These skeletal changes produce a shorter thorax with increased anterior–posterior diameter. In severe cases, the rib cage may rest on the pelvic bones that cause marked limitation of thoracic movement. The geriatric patient has no change in the partial pressure of carbon dioxide (CO_2). Consequently, elderly patients, who have a subtle decrease in their ability to deliver oxygen to the tissues, are more susceptible to retaining CO_2 or CO_2 narcosis, especially after being medicated for postoperative pain.

CARDIOVASCULAR

Elderly patients in general have higher blood pressures caused by decreased arterial elasticity, increasing peripheral vascular resistance and cardiac workload. Baroreceptors in the aorta and carotid arches become less sensitive to pressure changes in the arterial system and cardiac muscles. When the older adult experiences symptomatic hypotension, these chemoreceptors are less responsive to the sympathetic response of beta-adrenergic stimulation. In turn, there is a decreased ability of the cardiovascular system to autoregulate by vasoconstriction preferentially shunting blood from the peripheral arteries to the heart, lungs, and brain in times of stress. In addition, there is progressive stiffening of the myocardium; the heart valves become thick and rigid as a result of sclerosis and fibrosis, compounding dysfunction that leads to reduced efficiency. The decrease in the elasticity of the arteries that are responsible for vascular changes to the heart, kidneys, and pituitary gland, with a simultaneous increase in the rigidity of the vessel walls and the narrowing of the arterial lumens, necessitates a greater force to pump blood through the vessels. Cardiac output and stroke volume decrease with aging as a result of decreased conduction velocity and a reduction in coronary blood flow. In surgical patients where there is cardiac compromise, early placement of a pulmonary artery catheter and aggressive management of hemodynamic parameters have improved surgical outcomes such as pain management [15].

NEUROLOGIC

As one ages, there may be changes in cognitive ability, memory, and data acquisition followed by a decrease in cerebral blood flow and a loss neurologic functioning. These physiologic changes may be exhibited as: concentration difficulties, short-term memory loss, distractibility, slowed reaction time, decreased speed of performance, and difficulty organizing information.

Thus the ability of the brain to rapidly process, coordinate, and react to stimuli is diminished. This may compromise further the level of consciousness and neurologic status of the geriatric patient, especially if the patient has been medicated for pain. There is clinical evidence to indicate an aged-related increase in pain threshold, altered pain quality, and diminished sensitivity to lower levels of noxious stimulation, but an increased response to higher intensity stimuli and reduced tolerance to strong pain. This, however, does not mean older adults experience less pain when they actually report it. One must remember that the older adult suffers from multiple disease states, increased frailty, and reduced physiologic reserves. Therefore, the elderly may present with confusion, aggression, restlessness, or fatigue, which may lead to misdiagnosis and delays in seeking appropriate pain management.

RENAL

Renal elimination depends on kidney perfusion, glomerular filtration, and urine acidity. The renal mass declines progressively, so that by the age of 65 years, there is a 30% to 40% loss of glomeruli. The glomerular filtration rate is decreased even further because of degenerative changes in the tubules of the remaining glomeruli. Consequently, the kidneys are less efficient in concentrating urine. If the older adult is taking diuretics, the normal creatinine may not represent the true value. The biologic half-life is affected by the degree of kidney function [16]. Renal elimination depends on kidney perfusion, glomeruli filtration, and urine acidity. Altered filtration and decreased plasma volume, which occur in dehydration, are common as one ages. This can be detrimental to the geriatric patient. For example, streptomycin or gentamycin may be nephrotoxic. Then, too, other drugs are ineffective in the presence of low creatinine clearance [16].

LIVER

The microsomal enzyme system of the liver is the primary site of drug metabolism or biotransformation. Research studies report differences in rates of metabolism as people age. There is, however, decreased blood flow to the liver from disease or aging that results in: decreased hepatic mass, decreased hepatic blood flow, decreased enzyme activity, decreased enzyme inductibility, and decreased hepatic clearance [16].

The half-life of the drug then is increased as a result of decreased hepatic clearance. Additionally, the duration of drug action also is determined by the hepatic rate. Slow metabolism means that the drug will remain in the body longer and produce a prolonged half-life.

PERIOPERATIVE PATIENT EDUCATION

Perioperative patient education spans the continuum of preoperative, intraoperative, postanesthesia, and postoperative teaching. Preoperative teaching begins in the surgeon's office, when the patient is scheduled for surgery. This teaching continues during the preadmission period to prepare the older adult for the day of surgery through discharge home. Each component of teaching should enhance and re-enforce subsequent perioperative education. Appropriate geriatric teaching strategies should be used in the perioperative setting. Keep instructions clear and simple, communicating with a lower tone of voice, slowly and respectfully. The environment should be a comfortable setting with few distractions. Important information that should be reviewed with the older adult includes:

- Clear, simple directions that detail where to report on the day of surgery
- Appropriate apparel
- Pain management goals
- Written educational instructions for the patient and caregiver (in large print that is easy to read)
- Offering a magnifying glass to aid in reading

DISCHARGE PLANNING

Discharge planning before the day of surgery is the key to successful surgical outcomes. According to Burden [17], successful postsurgery discharge planning relies on:

- Comprehensive preoperative assessment
- Effective communication among the hospital or facility's caregivers, the physician's office, the patient, and the family
- Consideration of the patient's preoperative status
- A strong patient and family education plan

The more detailed and comprehensive the information gleaned from the preoperative assessment is, the better prepared the discharge plan will be. Identifying special needs such as home care needs, care of the family pet, and transportation helps the patient plan for a safe recovery. Questions to ask are listed in Box 4.

DAY OF SURGERY PREOPERATIVE PREPARATION

When the older adult is admitted to the hospital or facility, it is important to note which family members or significant others are in attendance. Foremost, if the older adult is having outpatient surgery, it is critical to establish that the

Box 4: Discharge planning checklist

Social support
- Does the patient live alone?
- Who will be with the patient? For how long?
- Ability of the caregiver?
- Who will drive the patient home?
- Does the patient provide primary care for another family member?
- Does the patient drive?

Home environment
- Does the home have stair steps?
- Is an elevator available?
- How far is the walk from the car to the inside of the house?
- What is the relationship of the bedroom, bathroom, and kitchen?
- Where is the telephone located?
- List of emergency contacts available by telephone
- Remove safety hazards: scatter rugs, small objects.
- Move cooking utensils to countertop as needed.
- Is there adequate food in the home?
- Clothing to wear on day of surgery for ease of undressing
- Entertainment sources: books, puzzles, television, movies, radio, crafts

Medical and surgery-related needs
- Supply of prescription medications: ongoing and surgery-specific
- Equipment needed for recovery: wheelchair, crutches, braces, cold packs,
- Wound-care supplies
- Follow-up physician appointment: data? transportation?

From Burden N. Discharge planning for the elderly ambulatory surgical patient. *JoPAN* *2004;*19(6):404; with permission.

geriatric patient has a responsible caregiver to provide home care and has arranged for postoperative transportation to home or to an extended care facility. Furthermore, establishing and documenting a mutually agreed date and time for the postoperative phone call ensure reliability that follow-up communication will occur.

The preoperative nursing assessment should validate all information that has been documented in the preadmission period on the patient's medical record. Patient identification and correct site surgery are vital and recognized patient safety goal priorities of care.

INTRAOPERATIVE NURSING CONSIDERATIONS

Intraoperative assessment involves validating all patient information during the interview in the preoperative unit or in the operating room (OR) holding area. Because this time period is considered one of the most stressful, the OR nurse must be attentive to every detail to ensure the following surgical care components are present and documented:

- Consent for surgery signed and witnessed
- Surgical site marked on body and verified in the medical record and on surgical schedule by attending surgeon of record

In addition, other critical information, such as fasting, whether dentures or partial plates have been removed, assessing for sensory aids (hearing aids or eye glasses), and canes or walkers, are important to note. Skin condition or skin breakdown, especially on the surgical site, is vital to inspect before positioning the patient on the operating table. Preparing the older adult concerning the operating environment helps decrease anxiety and increases coping mechanisms. After the preoperative assessment and teaching have been completed and documented, the OR nurse collaborates with the anesthesiologist to assure surgical readiness. Once the patient is transferred to the OR, it is important that the OR nurse remains in visual, tactile, or voice contact with the awake geriatric patient. If possible, allow the elderly to keep sensory aids (hearing aid) or dentures. Remembering to keep sound, especially one's voice to a minimum and avoiding laughter ensures professionalism and caring. Maintaining normothermia in the older adult in the cold OR environment is challenging. The OR nurse should be watchful to ensure correct positioning on the OR bed, changing positions slowly and gently. In addition, the elderly patient's skin is protected through the use of special pads so that pressure ulcers are prevented. The JCAHO patient safety initiative of time-out with the attending surgeon, anesthesiologist or nurse anesthetist, and circulating nurse is validated with the surgical and anesthesia team to ensure the right patient, right procedure, right site [18].

POSTOPERATIVE ASSESSMENT AND MANAGEMENT

The postanesthesia care unit (PACU) nurse must be vigilant in providing transitional care from a totally anesthetized patient to one who is fully alert or returned to baseline status. The PACU nurse employs critical thinking skills when assessing and managing the older adult recovering from anesthesia and surgery. The report from the anesthesia provider is vital to establishing baseline assessment parameters and the intraoperative course the geriatric patient encountered to compare PACU clinical findings and hemodynamic trends that occur. In addition, the systematic prioritization of the admission and ongoing assessments are critical to prudent nursing care. The PACU nurse uses this review of systems always beginning with:

- Airway
- Breathing/pulse oximetry

- Circulation/cardiac
- Neurologic
- Pain and comfort
- Hydration
- Muscular strengths in all extremities

Assessing mental status may be complicated if the patient has a history of dementia. The stir-up regime is performed every 15 minutes. The PACU nurse asks the recovering patient to take a deep breath and cough, and bend their knees up and down on the stretcher. This stimulates the patient to alertness and promotes circulation in arthritic extremities. The patient then is prepared better for transfer to the inpatient unit, phase II recovery, or home.

Managing pain in the older adult may be challenging. In acute pain management, opioids are the standard of care in the PACU. Dosing of opioids can be achieved simply in the elderly by starting with short-acting opioids and rapidly switching to controlled-released formulas with the emphasis on regular dosing rather than prn dosing. The PCA and PCEA therapeutic modalities promote more frequent dosing with lower doses of opioids. This provides better pain relief. Nonopioids also may be used in acute pain management. Prudent postanesthesia pain management for the older adult includes:

- Begin with lower doses and titrate upward.
- Combine lower doses of one or more agents to minimize dose-limiting adverse effects of monotherapy.
- Give medications on a regular basis to promote continuous analgesia.
- Integrate carefully titrated medications with nonpharmacologic strategies such as guided imagery and relation techniques.

Multi-approach treatment options should be employed when managing the older person's pain and comfort. It is important to communicate the geriatric patient's pain management information with colleagues. It is important for the postanesthesia nurse to believe reports of pain and promote patients' functional outcomes and quality of life.

DISCHARGE CONSIDERATIONS

Discharging the same-day surgery older adult requires the PACU nurse to ensure the geriatric patient and the family or caregiver are prepared to care for the patient in the home setting properly. Written discharge instructions should be reviewed with the patient and family carefully. Demonstrations for wound/procedure care should be given with the patient giving a return performance. Emergency telephone numbers should be listed on the discharge instruction forms. Signs and symptoms of infections are important for the patient and family to recognize and report to the doctor. The home should be prepared for the older adult who is recovering at home to prevent falls or injuries (See Box 4) [17].

It is vital to establish preoperatively that the elderly patient will receive a post-discharge phone call as a means to follow-up on the patient's recovery progress. Communication through the postoperative phone call may be problematic for the older adult. The patient may be unable to hear the telephone or not able to get the telephone in time because of limited mobility after surgery. Encouraging the family or caregiver to call the next morning to the same-day surgery center is another way to ensure follow-up is attained.

SUMMARY

Perioperative care of the older adult requires the specialized knowledge of the physiology of aging and the effects of surgery and anesthesia. Comprehensive nursing care planning is essential to providing safe nursing care throughout the perioperative continuum. Discharge teaching is vital to positive surgical outcomes. Finally, respecting the older adult as a unique individual promotes mutual understanding and coping strategies in a stressful surgical environment.

References

[1] Atwell D, Mossad EB. Preoperative anesthesia evaluation. In: Estafanous PG, Barash JG, Reves JG, editors. Cardiac anesthesia principles and clinical practice. 2nd edition. Philadelphia: Lippincott-Williams-Wilkins; 2002. p. 155–6.

[2] Jansen P. Care of the older patient. In: Swearingen PL, editor. All-in-one care planning resource. St. Louis (MO): 2004, Mosby; 2004. p. 101–14.

[3] Anderson MA. Caring for older adults holistically. 3rd edition. Philadelphia: FA Davis; 2003.

[4] Asher ME. Surgical considerations in the elderly. J Perianesth Nurs 2004;19(6):406–14.

[5] Koehle MM. Special needs of the older adult. In: Burden N, et al, editors. Ambulatory surgical nursing. 2nd edition. Philadelphia: WB Saunders; 2000. p. 643–71.

[6] Phillips N. Perioperative geriatrics. In: Philips N, editor. Berry & Kohn's operating room technique. St Louis (MO): Mosby; 2004. p. 155–77.

[7] Drain CB. Postanesthesia nursing: a critical care approach. 4th edition. Philadelphia: Elsevier; 2003.

[8] Saufl NM. Preparing the older adult for surgery and anesthesia. J Perianesth Nurs 2004;19(6):372–8.

[9] Pasternak LR. Does routine testing affect outcome? In: Fleisher LA, editor. Evidence-based practice of anesthesiology. Philadelphia: WB Saunders; 2004. p. 11–5.

[10] Dzankic S, et al. The prevalence and predictive value of abnormal laboratory tests in elderly surgical patients. Anesth Analg 2001;93:301–8.

[11] Kuchta A, Golembiewski J. Medication use in the elderly patient. J Perianesth Nurs 2004;19(6):415–24.

[12] Emergency Nurses Association. Trauma nursing core course instructor manual. 5th edition. Park Ridge (IL): Emergency Nurses Association; 2000. p. 151–9.

[13] Eliopoulos C. Adjustments in aging. In: Eliopoulos C, editor. Gerontological nursing. 4th edition. Philadelphia: Lippincott-Williams-Wilkins; 2001.

[14] Victor K. Properly assessing pain in the elderly. RN Magazine 2001;5:45–9.

[15] Beck LH. The aging kidney: defending a delicate balance of fluid and electrolytes. Geriatrics 2000;4:26–32.

[16] Wertheim WA. Review of two guidelines for assessing older adults. Geriatrics 2000;7: 61–6.

[17] Burden N. Discharge planning for the elderly ambulatory surgical patient. J Perianesth Nurs 2004;19(6):401–5.

[18] Watters JM. The elderly surgical patient. In: ACS surgery principles and practice, Available at: www.medscape.com/viewarticle/508534.

Nurs Clin N Am 41 (2006) 329–337

NURSING CLINICS
OF NORTH AMERICA

INDEX

Note: Page numbers of article titles are in **boldface** type.

0029-6465/06/$ – see front matter
doi:10.1016/S0029-6465(06)00036-3

Changing Your Address?

Make sure your subscription changes too! When you notify us of your new address, you can help make our job easier by including an exact copy of your Clinics label number with your old address (see illustration below.) This number identifies you to our computer system and will speed the processing of your address change. Please be sure this label number accompanies your old address and your corrected address—you can send an old Clinics label with your number on it or just copy it exactly and send it to the address listed below.

We appreciate your help in our attempt to give you continuous coverage. Thank you.

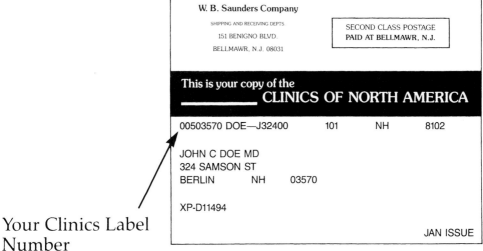

Your Clinics Label Number

Copy it exactly or send your label along with your address to:
Elsevier Periodicals Customer Service
6277 Sea Harbor Drive
Orlando, FL 32887-4800
Call Toll Free 1-800-654-2452

Please allow four to six weeks for delivery of new subscriptions and for processing address changes.